BREAST CANCER DIAGNOSIS

BREAST CANCER DIAGNOSIS

Gerald S. Johnston and A. Eric Jones

Department of Nuclear Medicine, Clinical Center
National Institutes of Health

PLENUM MEDICAL BOOK COMPANY • *New York and London*

Library of Congress Cataloging in Publication Data

Main entry under title:

Breast cancer diagnosis.

Includes bibliographical references and index.
1. Breast—Cancer—Diagnosis. 2. Radioisotope scanning. I. Johnston, Gerald S.,
1930-   II. Jones, Alfred Eric, 1935-   [DNLM: 1. Breast neoplasms—
Diagnosis. 2. Radioisotope scanning. 3. Mammography. WP870 B826]
RC280.B8B68   616.9'94'49   75-31980
ISBN 0-306-30893-2

Plenum Publishing Corporation
227 West 17th Street, New York, N. Y. 10011

United Kingdom edition published by Plenum Publishing Company, Ltd.
Davis House (4th Floor), 8 Scrubs Lane, Harlesden, London, NW10 6SE, England

Plenum Medical Book Company is an imprint of Plenum Publishing Corporation

Printed in the United States of America

CONTRIBUTORS

National Institutes of Health, Bethesda, Maryland

George S. Flinn, M.D.
Department of Radiology, Clinical Center

Robert S. Frankel, M.D.
Department of Nuclear Medicine, Clinical Center

Robert S. Francis, M.D.
Department of Radiology, Clinical Center

Gerald S. Johnston, M.D.
Department of Nuclear Medicine, Clinical Center

Alfred E. Jones, M.D.
Department of Nuclear Medicine, Clinical Center

James N. Ingle, M.D.
Medical Oncology, Medicine Branch
National Cancer Institute

Stanley M. Levenson, M.D.
Department of Nuclear Medicine, Clinical Center

Steven D. Richman, M.D.
Department of Nuclear Medicine, Clinical Center

Douglass C. Tormey, M.D., Ph.D.
Medical Oncology, Medicine Branch,
National Cancer Institute

PREFACE

Breast carcinoma is a dreaded disease. The incidence of breast cancer, which appears to be increasing, is 1 in 1500 women with an annual death rate of 4,000 from this disease in the United States (1). It is a cancer which threatens its victims with mutilation as well as early death. Although response to therapy has not been good, improved methods for earlier and more complete diagnosis are providing hope for better results.

When a woman presents herself for routine breast examination, what diagnostic procedures are indicated? If a breast mass is present, what diagnostic and therapeutic methods are employed? When the mass proves to be malignant, what then? Should biopsy and mastectomy be a combined procedure? Should a positive biopsy be followed by a complete diagnostic work-up before definitive therapy is undertaken? While some answers may seem obvious and others less obvious, common medical practices vary considerably in response to all of these situations. No easy formula exists. Each patient must be given individual consideration and her* treatment carefully planned to incorporate all the diagnostic findings. Experience to date indicates that some diagnostic and therapeutic procedures have established efficacy while others are not very helpful and still others need more evaluation before their usefulness can be assessed fully.

Traditionally, treatment of breast cancer has been surgical. Through the years poor results from surgery, along with acquisition of knowledge of the lymphatic spread of this malignancy, prompted more and more extensive surgical procedures. In the 1890's Halsted developed the radical mastectomy which then became a main surgical treatment for breast cancer (2). The 1940's saw the introduction of both radiation therapy and hormonal manipulations as therapeutic augmentations to surgery. Chemotherapy was added in the 1960's and continues to be developed in the 1970's. More conservative surgical modifications away from the Halsted procedure have been coming into vogue, and the place of radiation therapy in association with surgery continues to be investigated. Since no treatment has been established as having clear-cut advantages, considerable controversy exists over a "best approach" to the diagnosis and treatment of breast cancer.

---

*1% of breast carcinomas occur in men

However, one point has been agreed upon. When treatment is
initiated, the stage to which the disease has progressed can be
correlated with the patient's prognosis. A growing concern has
developed for earlier and earlier diagnosis so that survival can be
improved. Diagnostic methods are being developed for use in helping
plan more rational treatment for breast cancer and for assessing the
results of such treatment. Such diagnostic methods also permit
breast cancer patients to be followed closely for evidence of
recurrent metastatic disease.

A revolution is underway in medicine. A particularly vigorous
facet of this revolution is concerned with breast cancer. The call
for a more rational approach to breast cancer diagnosis and therapy
is being joined by those with the greatest commitment, women (3)
who have or may develop the disease.

In this volume, a review is presented of current diagnostic
methods with emphasis on the place of nuclear medical imaging as
applied to breast carcinoma. A reasonable diagnostic and therapeutic
approach to the patient is presented along with an assessment of the
expected yield from the wide range of potential tests. Generally,
these tests are innocuous and it is tempting to over use them.
However, only those with a strong liklihood of contributing to the
patient's diagnosis and care should be performed. In the instance
of mammography, the relatively high radiation exposure is also a
consideration for limiting the application of this useful procedure.

Permission to use these patient studies and x-rays was
generously granted by Dr. John L. Doppman, Chief, Department of
Radiology, Clinical Center and Dr. Douglass C. Tormey, Medical
Oncology Section, Medicine Branch National Cancer Institute.

Dr. Stanley Levenson, Mae F. Go, Dr. Julie E. Timins helped in
preparation of the manuscript. All scintigraphs were obtained with
the expert technical help of Janice H. Bird, Camille L. Boyce,
Elizabeth L. Evans, Eung T. Lee, Eleanor J. Myers and Sybil J.
Swann. The manuscript was typed by Phyllis E. Metzger, with the
assistance of Luella Bentz, and Paula K. McPherson.

(1)   Seidman, H. Cancer of the breast: statistical and epidemio-
      logical data. Cancer, 24: 1355, 1969.

(2)   Halsted, W.S. The results of radical operations for the cure
      of cancer of the breast. Ann Surg. 46: 80, 1907.

(3)   Kushner, R. Breast cancer. Harcourt, Brace, Jovanovich, New
      York, 1975.

CONTENTS

CHAPTER 1

Diagnostic Considerations in Breast Cancer

Douglass C. Tormey, M.D., Ph.D.
James N. Ingle, M.D.
Medical Oncology, Medicine Branch
National Cancer Institute
National Institutes of Health
Bethesda, Maryland

The breast is the most common site of female malignancy in the
United States, with carcinoma of the breast the leading cause of
mortality due to cancer in women between the ages of 15-74 years
(1). In the age group, 40-44, breast cancer is responsible for more
deaths than all other causes (2). The American Cancer Society
estimates that 90,000 women were diagnosed as having breast cancer
and 32,000 women died of the disease during 1974.

The most important prognostic factor at the time of
presentation is the extent of disease. A reduction in early
fatality rates was noted in patients screened periodically with
clinical examination and mammography (3). It would be desirable to
extend the concepts of earlier diagnosis and appropriate treatment
to all breast cancer patients, regardless of their disease stage.

Since there are no universal guidelines for the evaluation and
follow-up of patients with suspected, primary, or metastatic
disease, this discussion will present our views and those in the
literature concerning diagnostic concepts and procedures. Emphasis
will be placed on nuclear medicine techniques. Three general
clinical settings will be considered: (A) the patient with a
suspicious breast lesion, (B) the patient with proven primary breast
cancer and, (C) the patient with recurrent or metastatic disease.

A. The Patient with a Breast Lesion
The patient with a breast mass, nipple discharge or some other
complaint should be evaluated in a manner dictated by the history
and physical examination. For example, in cases of nipple
discharge, cytologic examination is indicated. Techniques are being
developed to obtain material from the nipple with a breast suction

pump and ductal cannulation. Those patients with a breast mass or suspicious skin changes should be evaluated with diagnostic procedures directed at further characterizing the breast lesion (Figure 1). As the sensitivity of the clinical examination is observer dependent, procedures such as mammography, xeroradiography, thermography and ultrasonotomography are utilized to improve diagnostic accuracy. When comparing clinical examination, mammography and thermography in 306 histologically confirmed breast cancers, the detection sensitivity of these modalities was 82%, 85%, and 72%, respectively (4). When clinical examination was combined with mammography, the accuracy increased to 92%. Ultrasonotomography, a relatively new procedure, has been reported capable of diagnosing breast cancer in 90% of cases (5); sensitivity for lesions less than 2 cms. was 82%. Breast scintigraphy, another modality, demonstrates 99mTc pertechnetate (6) and 67Ga localization in malignant breast tumors. Unfortunately, a significant incidence of false-positive and false-negative studies occur. This latter technique is fully discussed in Chapter 4. Of the aforementioned ancillary procedures, the mammogram is used most commonly and is discussed in Chapter 7 (Roentgenographic and Other Procedures).

In those patients with a high clinical suspicion of malignancy, an adequate histologic tissue specimen is necessary. Needle biopsy and needle aspiration are ideal procedures for this in view of their simplicity and low morbidity; neither appears to adversely affect patient survival (7,8). If either of these techniques is positive for malignancy, the patient should be fully evaluated for metastatic disease prior to definitive surgery (Table 1, Column 3). Essentially the same format is required in patients with a negative needle aspirate prior to biopsy under general anesthesia, followed by definitive surgery if the biopsy is positive (Table 1, Column 2). However, if the biopsy is performed several days prior to mastectomy, the extensive diagnostic testing can be postponed until biopsy results return (Table 1, Column 1). Table 1 does not include those studies performed on a routine pre-operative basis for the evaluation of cardiac, renal, metabolic and coagulation status. The importance of this preliminary evaluation is paramount, for the presence of metastatic disease dramatically alters therapy. Local surgical intervention may be modified and some form of systemic therapy instituted at an earlier date.

In these settings, patient evaluation is based upon the location of known metastatic disease. The distribution for disease sites varies among the literature. In one autopsy series, the major sites of metastases were: lung (77%); bone (75%); mediastinal lymph nodes (66%); pleura (65%); liver (61%); adrenals (54%); peritoneal and retroperitoneal lymph nodes (44%); pericardium (35%); brain (29%); peritoneum (25%); diaphragm (25%) and ovaries (23%) (9). For the purpose of planning a diagnostic protocol, however, of utmost

TABLE 1

DIAGNOSTIC PROCEDURES IN PATIENTS WITH SUSPECTED OR PROVEN PRIMARY BREAST CARCINOMA

Procedures	Prebiopsy Diagnosis Unknown	Preoperative Diagnosis Unknown	Preoperative Post Biopsy Diagnosis Cancer
History	x	x	x
Physical Examination	x	x	x
Mammogram or Xeroradiograph	x	x	x
CBC	x	x	x
Alkaline Phosphatase		x	x
SGOT or SGPT, Bilirubin		x	x
Chest X-ray		x	x
Needle Aspiration of Breast	x		
Biopsy of Breast Lesion	x		
Bone Scan		x	x
X-rays of Abnormal Areas on Bone Scan		x	x
Liver Scan		x^1	x^1
Brain Scan		x^2	x^2

[1] If abnormality of liver on physical examination or function tests
[2] If indicated by clinical abnormality

importance is the anatomic region of first recurrence. A study of
305 post-radical mastectomy patients, with and without three days of
post-operative chemotherapy, demonstrated the following statistical
distribution of first recurrence sites: integument (31%); skeletal
(26%); respiratory (19%); lymphatic (13%); digestive (9%); ovaries
(1%); and brain (1%) (10). Data for the groups were comparable,
with the exception of a slightly lower incidence of skeletal
metastases (21%) in the group not receiving chemotherapy. The
necessity for a thorough evaluation of these systems and organs is
then quite apparent.

Of critical interest, both prognostically and therapeutically
in any patient with a breast lesion, is the skeletal examination.
Advocated by many, with some variations, a skeletal survey
consisting of a lateral skull view, A-P and lateral radiographs of
the thoraco-lumbar spine, as well as A-P pelvic images could be
performed. The entire radiographic approach employed at the
National Institues of Health is described in Chapter 7. Suffice it
to say, the plain X-ray is considered an insensitive procedure for
evaluating these major sites of osseous metastases (11).

Bone scintigraphy, in contrast, has been found superior to
roentgenographic procedures by numerous investigators. A review of
the literature is presented in Chapter 5 (Skeletal Scintigraphy).
Controversy, however, still exists concerning the value of routine
pre-operative bone scanning and the metastatic survey. Robbins
reported in 1972 (12) and reiterated in 1974 (13), that these
procedures are indicated only in patients with bone pain, or when a
primary lesion greater than 5 cms. in diameter is accompanied by
extensive axillary metastases. This contention was based on the
analysis of over 300 potentially curable breast cancer patients, of
whom only 19% developed osseous metastases within 10 years of their
primary surgery. The justification for these techniques would be
their utility in the decision for mastectomy.

Contradictory information was obtained by Galasko (14), who
evaluated fluorine-18 bone scintigraphy in 50 pre-operative patients
with breast carcinoma. In no instance was metastatic disease
detectable either clinically or radiologically. Radiographs of the
lateral skull, as well as cervical, thoracic, lumbar spine, and P-A
pelvis were obtained. Primary tumors ranged in size from less than
2 cms. to larger than 5 cms. in their greatest dimension. All
patients had either no palpable ipsilateral axillary nodes or
movable ipsilateral axillary lymph nodes. Twelve (24%) were found
to have bone scan abnormalities suggestive of metastatic disease.
Lesions in 10 of these 12 patients were subsequently visualized
roentgenographically or confirmed at autopsy. No correlation was
made between primary tumor size, nodal status and bone scan
findings.

Current evidence would suggest the use of bone scanning in preference to the roentgenographic survey in a patient with suspected carcinoma of the breast prior to biopsy and definitive surgery. While the yield may be low, potentially significant baseline images are available for future reference. Gerber et al. (15) reported a 5% incidence of positive pre-operative 99mTc diphosphonate bone scans in 109 patients with Stage I or II breast carcinoma. During the 3-24 month post-operative period, follow-up studies in 48 women demonstrated scan conversion from normal to abnormal in 11 (23%). Of this group, 73% were post-menopausal. Both pre-operative baseline and serial post-operative bone scanning were recommended. If a scintigraphic abnormality is discovered, roentgenographic correlation is advisable. In cases of a positive bone scan with negative roentgenograms, tomography will frequently demonstrate disease. The thoroughness of this approach has provided sites for bone biopsy, thus establishing a definitive diagnosis.

In evaluating the liver, routine biochemical tests include alkaline phosphatase, bilirubin, SGOT and SGPT. There is disagreement concerning the indications for liver scanning. It is well accepted that in the patient with a known malignancy, the liver scan can provide visible evidence for metastases. This is most often observed in the presence of abnormal liver function tests and/or hepatomegaly. Still in question is the value of liver scintigraphy in the presence of normal liver function tests and physical examination. Poulose et al. (16), in an evaluation of a variety of primary neoplasms, recommended liver scanning prior to major tumor surgery in every patient, including those with unremarkable physical and biochemical hepatic findings. Excluding the bromsulphalein (BSP) dye test, 33% of 54 patients with hepatic metastases demonstrated as many as four normal biochemical liver function tests. In addition, livers of normal size were noted in 54% of 104 necropsy patients with metastatic liver disease. In contrast, Rosenthal and Kaufman (17) reported nine false-negative scans in 10 patients with documented liver metastases; liver function tests and hepatic examination were normal. In 62 other patients with no evidence for secondary neoplasm, the scan was falsely abnormal or equivocal in seven. Biochemical and clinical parameters were again normal.

While the sensitivity of this procedure relative to biochemical tests and physical examination may prove a valuable baseline procedure, routine liver scintigraphy in patients with suspected breast cancer has not been rewarding. The experience and approach in our protocol setting is described in Chapter 2 (Liver Scintigraphy).

Brain scanning, while a useful tool in the detection and confirmation of cerebral metastases, is indicated only in the

TABLE 2

PERCENT RECURRENCE RATES IN BREAST CANCER PATIENTS
ACCORDING TO IPSILATERAL AXILLARY LYMPH NODE STATUS
AT TIME OF MASTECTOMY

Nodes		Time After Mastectomy		
Status	Number	18 Months	5 Years	10 Years
Negative	–	5%	21%	24%
Positive	1-3	16%	49%	65%
Positive	>3	44%	81%	86%

presence of neurological signs or symptoms. Although Quinn
described the excellent sensitivity of brain scanning in 32 of 34
patients with proven intracerebral breast metastases (18), its value
as a routine screening agent in our patient population has not been
demonstrated (Chapter 3, Brain Scintigraphy).

Whole body 67Ga scanning has also been studied in breast
cancer. Richman et al. (19), retrospectively evaluated the utility
of 67Ga scintigraphy in 125 primary and metastatic breast carcinoma
patients (Chapter 6). With rare exception, this scintigraphic
procedure demonstrated only corroborative capabilities and was
inferior to individual organ tracer studies. Gallium-67
scintigraphy is not recommended in the absence of metastatic
disease.

    B. Proven Primary Breast Cancer
The goal of the post-operative follow-up program is to detect
disease recurrence at the earliest possible date. The intensity of
this program should be determined by the risk of recurrence. At the
present time, ipsilateral axillary nodal status at mastectomy
appears to be the most reliable single prognostic indicator. Fisher
et al. (20,21) have classified the lymph node status of these
patients as follows: (1) negative nodes, (2) 1 to 3 positive nodes,
and (3) greater than 3 positive nodes. The recurrence rates of
these groups of patients are markedly different (Table 2).

With these considerations, a follow-up program is proposed in
Tables 3 and 4. For the first five years following mastectomy,
intensive efforts are undertaken to detect recurrent or metastatic
disease (Table 3); in the ensuing 5-10 years (Table 4), the
follow-up program can usually be relaxed. Although the majority of
patients with positive axillary lymph nodes at the time of
mastectomy demonstrate recurrence within the first five
post-operative years, a significant number will also relapse during
the second five year period. Since patients with negative lymph
nodes have a low recurrence rate during the 5 to 10 year period,
bone scans and chest roentgenograms can probably be eliminated as
routine procedures in this group. The determining factor in these
situations remains at the physician's discretion. After 10 years
patients will continue to relapse, but most can probably be followed
with an annual history, physical examination and blood studies as
noted in Table 3. In those women with a history of positive
axillary nodes, yearly chest roentgenograms and bone scans are
suggested. Ideally, all follow-up programs should minimize
inconvenience, discomfort and psychological stress to the patient,
without sacrificing an early diagnosis of recurrence.

Concerning the asymptomatic patient, roentgenograms should be
performed after identification of abnormal areas on bone scan.

TABLE 3

POSTOPERATIVE FOLLOW-UP OF PATIENTS WITH NO EVIDENCE OF

RESIDUAL CANCER DURING THE FIRST FIVE YEARS AFTER MASTECTOMY

(Intervals in Months)

	Negative Nodes	Positive Nodes	
		1 to 3	>3
History	6	3 to 6	3
Physical Examination	6	3 to 6	3
CBC	12	6	3
SGOT or SGPT	12	6	3
Alkaline Phosphatase	12	6	3
Chest X-ray	12	6	3
Bone Scan	12	6	3

TABLE 4

FOLLOW-UP PROGRAM FOR PATIENTS WITH NO EVIDENCE OF RESIDUAL

CANCER FROM FIVE TO TEN YEARS AFTER MASTECTOMY

(Intervals in Months)

	Negative Nodes	Positive Nodes	
		1 to 3	>3
History	6	6	6
Physical Examination	6	6	6
CBC	12	12	12
SGOT or SGPT	12	12	12
Alkaline Phosphatase	12	12	12
Chest X-ray	-	12	12
Bone Scan	-	12	12

Liver and brain scans do not appear to be effective screening tests
for recurrent disease and need only be performed if clinically
indicated. Although the patient with a history of cancer in one
breast is at higher risk of developing cancer in the other breast
than the general population, this occurs at a relatively low rate of
1% per year. Routine mammography should probably be reserved for
select high risk patients, such as those with a more aggressive type
of primary disease.

Biochemical tumor marker studies are also of interest in
patients with proven primary breast cancer. While still in the
preliminary stages of evaluation, elevated serum carcinoembryonic
antigen (CEA) values were noted in several cases of resected,
apparently localized primary carcinoma of the breast (22,23).
Although non-specific, these findings may suggest this test as
potentially more sensitive than conventional diagnostic modalities.

C. Recurrent or Metastatic Disease

Once the patient has disseminated disease, the frequency of
follow-up is increased. This course is chosen to ascertain
treatment failures with dispatch. Hopefully, more effective therapy
can then be instituted. The frequency of these procedures is
directly related to the types of therapy. For example, a complete
blood count may be obtained once a month with hormonal therapy, but
weekly intervals would be more preferable with some combination
chemotherapy regimens. A basic follow-up program is outlined in
Table 5.

Regarding imaging procedures for skeletal evaluation, the bone
scan provides greater sensitivity in the detection of new lesions,
while skeletal roentgenograms are more sensitive for following sites
of known disease. Concepts concerning diagnostic imaging procedures
in patients with skeletal metastases are elaborated upon in Chapter
5 (Skeletal Scintigraphy).

Other tests have a variable degree of utility in the follow-up
evaluation of metastatic breast disease. The liver scan, when
abnormal, rarely contributes significantly to patient management
unless a lesion of greater than 5 cms. is present (24). Despite
these limitations, a baseline liver scan in the patient with known
metastatic disease is recommended. This may provide useful
information should the patient subsequently develop abnormalities in
liver function tests or physical examination. Irregularities by
either of these parameters warrants liver scintigraphy. When
metastases are demonstrated, progressive disease and response to
therapy can be evaluated. Baseline or routine brain scanning
without neurological manifestations is not advocated in this
clinical setting. It has been our experience that this procedure
does not provide significant information. Gallium-67 scanning, as

TABLE 5

FOLLOW-UP INTERVALS IN PATIENTS WITH

METASTATIC CARCINOMA OF THE BREAST

Test	Intervals (Weeks)
History	1-4
Physical Examination	1-4
CBC	1-4
SGOT or SGPT	4
Alkaline Phosphatase	4
Chest X-ray	8-12
Bone Scan	12
X-rays of abnormal areas being monitored and new abnormalities on bone scan	12

previously noted, rarely contributes to the data gained by other
modalities. However, it has been more sensitive than mediastinal
tomography in detecting mediastinal lesions in several cases (19)
(Chapter 6). Whole body 67Ga scintigraphy is not presently
recommended as a routine test. Mammography also seldom provides
objectively measurable parameters. A bone marrow biopsy may be
helpful for guiding the use of chemotherapy, although its value in
follow-up is unknown. As a diagnostic tool in breast cancer
patients, however, it is considerably more sensitive than a bone
marrow aspirate (25). A BSP test is potentially useful if other
liver function tests are normal, although its importance in
follow-up could be lessened by the effects of chemotherapy. The
value of tumor markers such as CEA, in the setting of metastatic
disease, has not been established; nevertheless, a favorable
clinical response was accompanied by a decrease in abnormally
elevated CEA levels in several breast cancer patients (22,25).

Of final note is the topic of estrogen receptor analysis, a
subject which applies to both primary and metastatic breast
carcinoma patients. This field of study has been comprehensively
covered in detail by McGuire et al. (26). Whenever tumor tissue is
available for biopsy, either prior to or during a therapeutic
maneuver, recent evidence suggests the advisability of submitting a
portion of the specimen for estrogen receptor analysis. Depending
upon the technique utilized, the assay can be performed with as
little as 10 mg. of tissue in most situations; however, 200-500 mgs.
of tissue are occasionally required. Suffice it to say, an
experienced laboratory is necessary.

The presence or absence of estrogen receptor binding protein
appears to have prognostic ramifications for the subsequent response
of the patient to various types of hormonal manipulation. Among the
modes of endocrine intervention are: adrenalectomy, oophorectomy,
and hypophysectomy, as well as exogenous therapy with estrogens,
androgens, or corticosteroids. If no estrogen receptor is present,
the probability of remission induction with these procedures is
5-10%. When the estrogen receptor protein is found, there is a
marked increase in the likelihood of response to either surgical or
exogenous hormonal therapy; 50-65% of this group have achieved
remission under these circumstances. At present, there is no
correlation between the estrogen receptor status (quantitatively or
qualitatively), the duration of the post-operative disease-free
interval, or the durability of any response obtained in metastatic
disease. Intensive efforts are continuing in this most interesting
field of study.

In summary, there are numerous approaches and modalities for
evaluating patients with a suspicious breast lesion, proven primary
breast cancer, and recurrent or metastatic disease. The nuclear

medicine procedure best serving these patients appears to be whole
body skeletal scintigraphy. Liver, brain and 67Ga scintigraphy
should be selectively applied to high risk patients and in those
situations where clinical or biochemical evidence is suggestive of
disease.

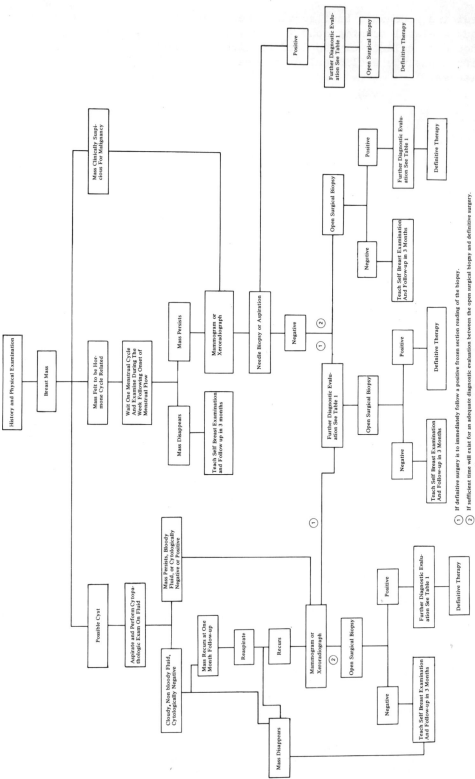

Fig. 1-1. Diagnostic flow in patients with a breast mass.

References Chapter 1

1. U. S. Public Health Service, National Vital Statistics
    Division: Vital Statistics of the United States, Annual
    1930-1968. Washington U. S. Government Printing Office,
    1934-71.

2. Silverberg, D., Holleb, A.I. Cancer Statistics - 1971.
    Cancer 21: 13, 1971.

3. Shapiro, S., Strax, P., Venet, L. Periodic breast cancer
    screening in reducing mortality from breast cancer. JAMA 215:
    1777, 1971.

4. Isard, H., Becker, W., Shilo, R., Ostrum, B. Breast
    thermography after four years and 10,000 studies. Amer J
    Roentgenol 115: 811, 1972.

5. Kobayashi, T., Takatani, O., Hattori, N., Kimura, K.
    Differential diagnosis of breast tumors. The sensitivity
    graded method of ultrasonotomography and clinical evaluation
    of its diagnostic accuracy. Cancer 33: 940, 1974.

6. Villarreal, R.L., Parkey, R.W., Bonte, F.J. Experimental per-
    technetate mammography. Radiology 111: 657, 1974.

7. Berg, J.W., Robbins, G.F. A late look at the safety of aspir-
    ation biopsy. Cancer 15: 826, 1962.

8. Robbins, G.F., Brothers, J.H., Eberhart, W.F., Quan, S. Is
    aspiration biopsy of breast cancer dangerous to the patient?
    Cancer 7: 774, 1954.

9. Abrams, H.L., Spiro, R., Goldstein, N. Metastases in
    carcinoma. Analysis of 1000 autopsied cases. Cancer 3: 74,
    1950.

10. Fisher, B., Ravdin, R.G., Ausman, R.K., Slack, N.H., Moore, G.E.,
    Noer, R.J. Surgical adjuvant chemotherapy in cancer of
    the breast: Results of a decade of cooperative investigation.
    Ann Surg 168: 337, 1968.

11. Edelstyn, G.A., Gillespie, P.J., Grebbell, F.S. The radio-
    logical demonstration of osseous metastases. Experimental
    observations. Clin Radiol 18: 158, 1967.

12. Robbins, G.F., Knapper, W.H., Barrie, J., Kripalani, I.,
    Lawrence, J. Metastatic bone disease developing in patients
    with potentially curable breast cancer. Cancer 29: 1702,
    1972.

13. Robbins, G.F. The rationale for the treatment of women with
     potentially curable breast carcinoma. Surg Clin North America
     54: 793, 1974.

14. Galasko, C.S.B. Skeletal metastases and mammary cancer. Ann
     Roy Coll Surg Engl 50: 3, 1972.

15. Gerber, F.H., Goodreau, J.J., Kirchner, P.T. Tc-99m-EHDP bone
     scanning in breast carcinoma. J Nucl Med 16: 529, 1975.

16. Poulose, K.P., Reba, R.C., Deland, F.H., Wagner, H.N. Role of
     liver scanning in the preoperative evaluation of patients with
     cancer. Brit Med J 4: 585, 1969.

17. Rosenthal, S., Kaufman, S. The liver scan in metastatic
     disease. Arch Surg 106: 656, 1973.

18. Quinn III, J.S. Use of diagnostic nuclear medicine procedures
     in breast cancer. Cancer 28: 1695, 1971.

19. Richman, S.D., Brodey, P.A., Frankel, R.S., De Moss, E.V.,
     Tormey, D.C. Johnston, G.S. Breast scintigraphy with
     99mTc pertechnetate and 67Ga citrate. J Nucl Med 16:
     293, 1975.

20. Fisher, B., Slack, N.H., Bross, I.D.J. Cancer of the breast:
     Size of neoplasm and prognosis. Cancer 24: 1071, 1969.

21. Fisher, B. A report to the profession from the Breast Cancer
     Task Force of the National Cancer Institute, Bethesda,
     Maryland, National Institutes of Health, September 30, 1974.

22. Steward, A.M., Nixon, D., Zamcheck, N., Aisenberg, A.
     Carcinoembryonic antigen in breast cancer patients: Serum
     levels and disease progress. Cancer 33: 1246, 1974.

23. Tormey, D.C., Waalkes, T.P., Ahmann, D., Gehrke, C.W.,
     Zumwatt, R.W., Snyder, J., Hansen, H. Biologic markers in
     breast carcinoma. I. Incidence of abnormalities of CEA, HCG,
     three polyamines, and three minor nucleosides. Cancer 35:
     1095, 1975.

24. Moertel, C. Personal communication.

25. Ingle, J., Tormey, D., Bull, J. Bone marrow involvement in
     breast cancer. Proceedings of the American Association for
     Cancer Research and of the American Society of Clinical
     Oncology. 16: 245, 1975.

26. McGuire, W.L., Carbone, P.P., Vollmer, E.P.(eds.) Estrogen
     receptors in human breast carcinoma. New York, Raven Press,
     1975.

CHAPTER 2

Liver Scintigraphy

Stanley Levenson, M.D.

Department of Nuclear Medicine
National Institutes of Health
Bethesda, Maryland

Liver scanning has become an integral part of the diagnosis and management of patients with secondary hepatic neoplasm. Its utility in breast cancer patients is therefore clearly apparent. Metastatic liver disease was present in 51% of cases at autopsy in a series collected by Meissner and Warren (1), ranking the liver along with nodal, lung and skeleton as one of the most frequent sites of secondary neoplasm. Fifteen to twenty percent of patients die as a result of hepatic decompensation with up to 50% having clinically significant involvement (2). Nemoto and Dao found a 38% incidence of liver metastasis in postmenopausal women at adrenalectomy and in 31% of premenopausal patients who underwent therapeutic oophorectomy (3).

Because of the extremely serious nature of this disease, it is crucial to have a noninvasive technique such as liver scanning to evaluate patients at the time of their diagnosis and initial therapy, and to provide an indicator for future follow-up. While visualizing metastatic disease in a clinically suspicious liver is foremost in the mind of the investigator, present-day inherent scanning limitations in the detection of secondary disease require that the lesion be at least 2 cms. in size for visualization (4-8). Special additional problems arise in breast carcinoma patients, because of the increasing popularity of chemotherapy as well as hormonal and local radiotherapy (9).

In addition, with an exclusively female patient population, hepatic related disorders, such as gallbladder disease, may present confusing hepatic defects mistaken for neoplasm (10, 11). An I-131

19

rose bengal liver scan assists in preventing false-positive
diagnoses (12).

It is therefore necessary to judiciously evaluate the liver scan
with all available parameters before diagnosing metastatic liver
disease. Just as in other patients with a predisposing primary
neoplasm, nonhomogeneous tracer distribution without discrete focal
filling defects should not be over-interpreted (13). Correlation of
suspicious scans with clinical hepatic enlargement or change in
hepatic size, as well as incorporation of blood chemistries such as
alkaline phosphatase and serum transaminase levels will invariably
enhance the diagnostic accuracy of this procedure. Without the
scan, abnormal liver function tests are non-specific and can be
quite misleading (18). It is well known, however, that metastatic
disease, in its own insidious fashion, may be unexpectedly detected
in the absence of physical or biochemical manifestations (18,19)
(Fig. 2-1). This should encourage heightened awareness on the part
of the clinician in young, premenopausal patients, and in those
women with a more highly malignant carcinoma, e.g., anaplastic
carcinoma. When studies appear equivocal, as they do in many cases,
the scintiscan may then be useful as a geographic parameter for
liver biopsy (5,12,18). If normal tissue is obtained, as occurs in
many patients with questionable, or limited but definite focal
disease, peritoneoscopy, using the liver scan as a guide, has been
rewarding (20). While hepatic angiography may also be employed
following a questionable scan (21,22), it is rarely used for
diagnosis in this patient population.

The liver scintigraphic technique that is routinely employed is
as follows: patients receive 2 mCi 99mTc sulfur colloid
intravenously. Scintiphotos are obtained approximately 10 minutes
post-injection in the anterior supine position with right and left
costal margin markers. The gamma camera, because of its flexibility
and large field of view, has been the instrument of choice for this
procedure. The remainder of the images are obtained in the upright
position, including a second anterior view which frequently
clarifies suspicious regions and provides information regarding
liver pliability (23). Right lateral and posterior views are
similarly performed, as well as corresponding images of the spleen.
Oblique views are obtained in questionable situations. In
evaluating the utility of liver scanning in our patient population,
scans were performed on a quarterly basis, and more frequently when
warranted by the clinical course. Over 600 liver scans were
obtained during the two year interval, January 1973 - January 1975.

The abnormalities detected in liver scintiscanning are numerous.
One must always be aware of artefacts   (10,24,25), and in
particular, those in the superior dome on the right lobe secondary
to an overlying breast, a breast prosthesis (26), or a portal of

radiation (5). This latter finding may also involve both right and left hepatic lobes after extensive irradiation to the thoracic spine. Rib margin indentations can also produce linear hepatic defects which usually assume the contour of the costal margin (5). All the above have been noted to cause generalized decreases in hepatic tracer in the aforementioned regions (Fig. 2-2).

Another not uncommon finding is flattening of the superior dome of the right hepatic lobe (Fig. 2-3). This is frequently, but not always, accompanied by an excessive extension of the liver beneath the right costal margin with palpatory findings indicating hepatomegaly. The presentation of a flattened dome and inferiorly displaced liver should always alert one to the possibility of a pleural effusion or chronic obstructive pulmonary disease as the etiology (27).

Undiagnosed or underlying liver disease can be extremely perplexing in scan interpretation, frequently causing varying degrees of tracer nonhomogeneity and hepatomegaly (5,28)(Fig. 2-4). Again, the imposing influence of a breast carcinoma diagnosis, particularly with bone and/or lymph node metastases, may incorrectly bias the scan interpretation. Hepatic abnormalities secondary to anesthesia induced toxic hepatitis incurred at the time of the patient's mastectomy, hepatic changes associated with systemic chemotherapeutic agents, and serum hepatitis resulting from blood transfusion, demonstrate acute and occasionally chronic changes in the scintiscan. Instances of hepatic fatty infiltration, focal fibrosis and inflammation (etiology unknown) and cirrhosis yield scan images, which in this milieu, would raise the probability of liver metastases. Strict criteria for focal defect interpretation and follow-up scans are suggested.

Liver scanning is also a useful adjunct in elucidating the progression of documented metastases (Figs. 2-5,6,7), and evaluating the response to chemotherapy (Fig. 2-8). While the former is appreciated quite frequently, resolution or significant improvement is also being seen more commonly. Hepatic scintigraphy is now a routine procedure in determining hepatic response to chemotherapy.

As with any form of metastatic liver disease, it is obligatory to evaluate both hepatic lobes. Although the right lobe is more frequently and extensively involved, most probably because of its size and vascularity, the diagnosis of occult disease in the left lobe can radically alter patient therapy (Fig. 2-9).

In certain instances, 67Ga citrate scanning has localized in "cold" areas visualized on the 99mTc sulfur colloid images.

Generally this has not proven to be the case; however, the finding appears to predominate with extensive disease. In the liver, as in other regions of the body, 67Ga has been suboptimal in selectively localizing lesions of metastatic breast carcinoma (Fig. 2-10).

Concerning the spleen, no correlation has been observed with the reported 12% incidence of splenic metastases at autopsy. While images of the spleen are routinely included with liver scintiscans, infiltrative splenic disease has not been visualized. Relative increases in splenic tracer concentration have been seen in patients with significant liver metastases, but, this is the expected finding in cases of severe hepatic compromise due to secondary neoplasm. Four cases of splenomegaly have been observed in our patient population; the etiology is unexplained, since in no instance was hepatic disease evident.

Regarding the sensitivity of liver scanning in patients with known metastatic breast carcinoma, a review of 27 histologically proven cases demonstrated the liver scan as the first index of disease in seven (26%) (30). Abnormal liver function studies and/or physical examination raised the clinician's suspicion in the remaining cases. In no instance was the scan normal in this study group. Other investigators have reported a detection accuracy of 77% in secondary hepatic breast carcinoma; this has been attributed to the interval progression or occurrence of disease between scanning and histopathological documentation, and to the in vivo detection limitations of present-day instrumentation (8).

In conclusion, 99mTc sulfur colloid liver scanning has been found to be an excellent tool in the evaluation of metastatic disease in breast carcinoma patients. It is recommended for the visual documentation of suspected disease, response to chemotherapy, assessing neoplastic progression, and in the presence of abnormal liver function tests, physical evidence for hepatomegaly, or both. Scintigraphic evidence of occult preoperative metastases at the time of presentation should also radically alter surgical plans. This information would then allow a planned approach to the treatment of liver secondaries. On a routine basis, liver scan abnormalities preceded biochemical and physical findings in a significant number of patients. The importance of earlier recognition of metastases and its effect on long-term survival in this age of combination chemotherapy has yet to be determined (31).

Fig. 2-1. At age 32, this patient underwent a right radical mastectomy for infiltrating adenocarcinoma for the breast. There were no positive axillary lymph nodes. A biopsy of the left breast also revealed malignant tissue. Serial studies beginning in July, 1973, demonstrate what appeared to be metastatic changes on February 15, 1974. Percutaneous and peritoneoscopic biopsies were not helpful.

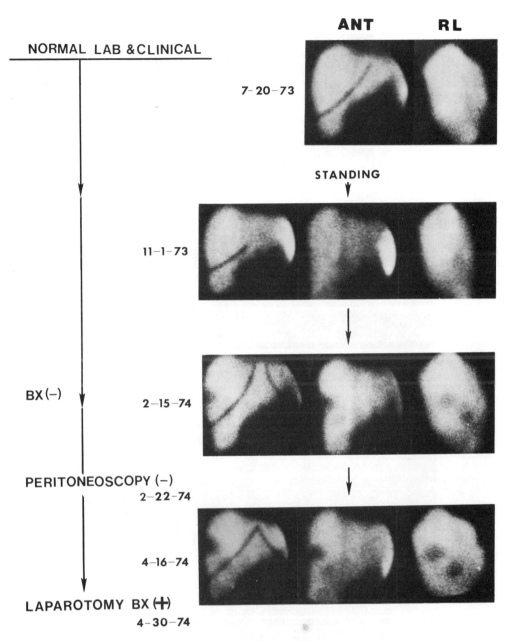

It was not until April 30, 1974, that a biopsy at laparotomy confirmed scan findings. This case exemplifies the detection of
metastatic disease by liver scan in the presence of normal liver
function tests, physical examination and multiple biopsy attempts.
(Ant = anterior reclining, standing = anterior upright, RL = right
lateral.)

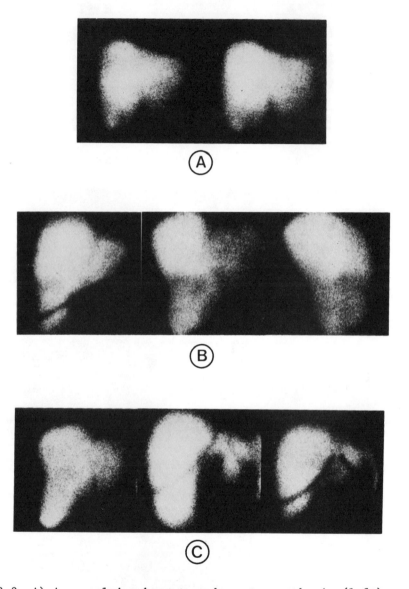

Fig. 2-2. A) An overlying breast or breast prosthesis (left) may
decrease the tracer concentration in the superior portion of the
right hepatic lobe. This is in contrast to the image in which the
artifact has been removed (right). B) Costal compression frequently
produces the linear defect seen here in the anterior supine, anterior
upright and right lateral projection. C) The pre-vertebral irradiation image (left) is followed by the scan demonstrating a midline
tracer decrease following irradiation (middle) and a resolving pattern over the next several months (right). Costal markers are in
place on the first scan in (B) and the 2nd and 3rd scans in (C).

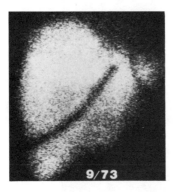
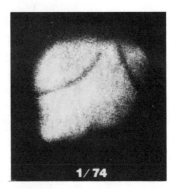
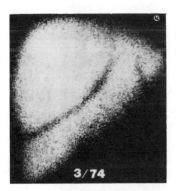
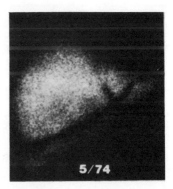

Fig. 2-3. A liver that was somewhat enlarged with nonhomogeneous tracer distribution by scan was followed serially for one year. Bone and bone marrow metastases were first documented in April, 1973, approximately four years after the patient's left radical mastectomy for carcinoma. Pleural effusion with negative cytology in June, 1973, demonstrated malignant cells in January, 1974. Note that the superior dome of the liver progresses from a flattened contour to its normal position and arch with resolution of the pleural fluid following thoracentesis and chemotherapy. Diaphragmatic flattening is also observed in patients with chronic obstructive pulomary disease.

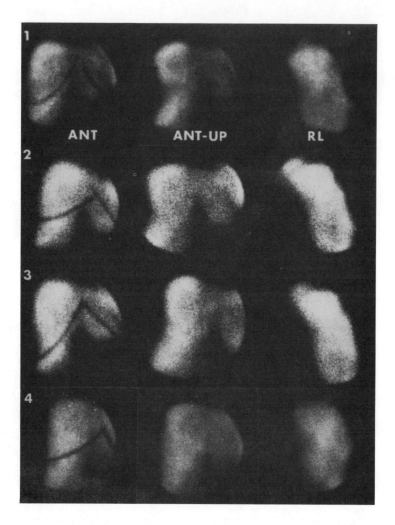

Fig. 2-4. Serial scintiphotos in a patient following her second
mastectomy for breast carcinoma demonstrate the potential for scan
over-interpretation in this population. The initial study (1) performed five months after mastectomy demonstrated hepatomegaly with
nonhomogeneous tracer distribution. The repeat study three months
later revealed minimal changes (2). The liver span was 17 cms. in
the mid-clavicular line with serum transaminase levels 5-25 times
normal. Eight months following the initial study, persistence of
the scan findings was noted (3), although enzymes were now normal
and the patient was well. Biopsy revealed acute hepatitis, which
in retrospect, was thought secondary to halothane toxicity at the
time of mastectomy. The final scan (4) obtained one year after the
original studies most likely reflects residual hepatic changes.
(Ant = anterior supine, Ant-up = anterior upright, RL = right
lateral.)

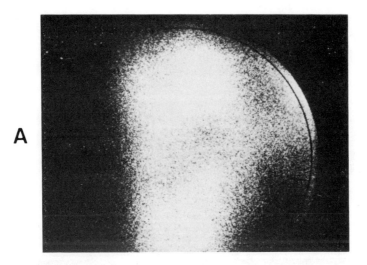

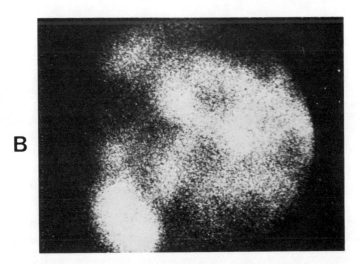

Fig. 2-5. Metastatic liver disease, first documented by scan three years post-radical mastectomy in November 1967, has been followed for almost five years. From 1970 (5A) through 1974 (5B), changes in hepatic scintiphotos have corresponded with the patient's liver function tests, physical findings and general well-being. This most unusual case provides exceptionally long-term followup and survival with severe secondary hepatic involvement.

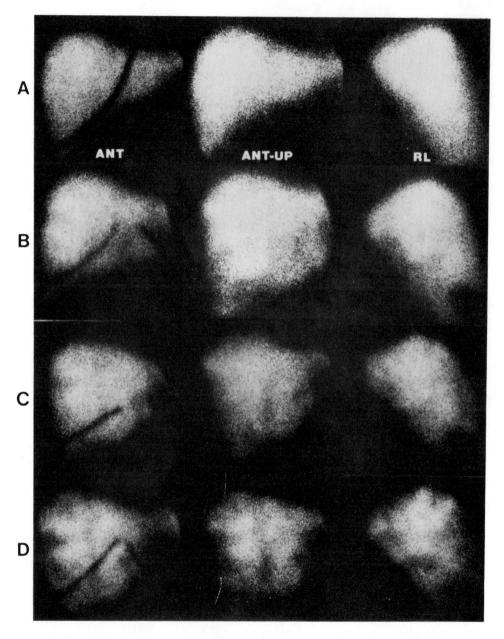

Fig. 2-6. Four liver scans over a one year interval demonstrate the
spectrum of appearance of secondary hepatic neoplasm. Normal (6A),
nonhomogeneous (6B), patchy (6C), and multiple focal defects
(6-D), describe the progressive temporal changes depicted above.
Clinical and biochemical parameters were of no assistance. (Ant =
anterior reclining, Ant-up = anterior upright, RL= right lateral).

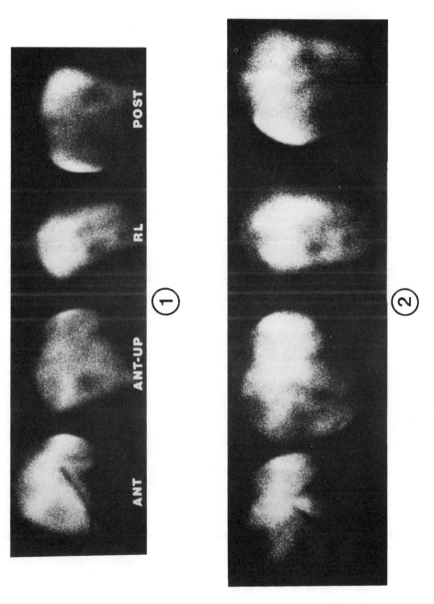

Fig. 2-7. Studies performed seven weeks apart (#1 and #2) demonstrate unusually agressive metastatic disease in a 29 year old post-mastectomy patient.

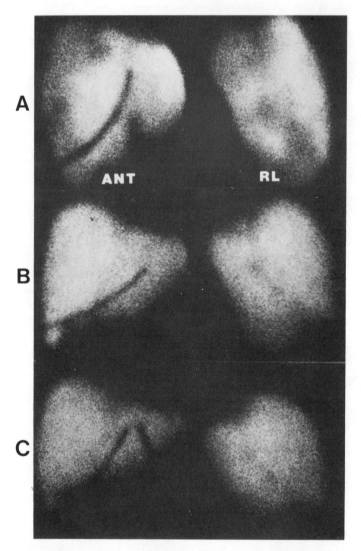

Fig. 2-8. The liver of this patient who has infiltrating ductal
cell carcinoma, demonstrates a remarkable response to chemotherapy.
Anterior and right lateral images performed initially (A), four (B)
and five (C) months following the initiation of therapy demonstrate
a dramatic temporal response to chemotherapy. The scan performed
after clinical evaluation (A) revealed an enlarging liver with
multiple focal filling defects almost certainly representing secondary hepatic neoplasm, although liver function studies were normal.
Sequential scans over the five month interval provided the clinician
with excellent documentation of the response to therapy in the presence of minimal physical findings and consistently normal liver
function text. (Ant = anterior reclining, RL = right lateral.)

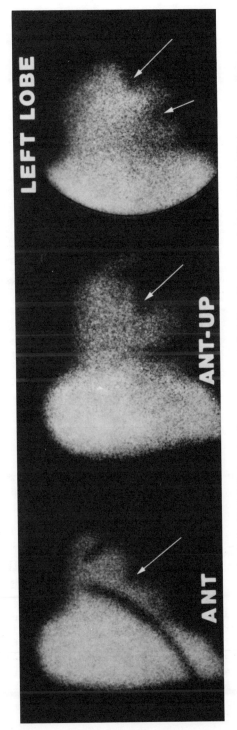

Fig. 2-9. Routine liver scanning in this patient revealed metastatic disease in the left lobe which was easily accessible to periotoneoscopic biopsy. The middle image was performed with the patient in the upright position (ant = anterior reclining, ant-up = anterior upright, left lobe = anterior view of left lobe.)

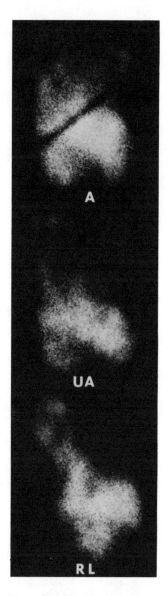
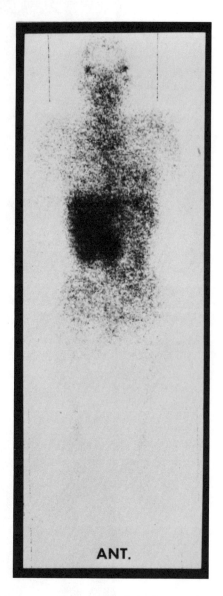

Fig. 2-10. Gallium-67 liver images have not been helpful in patients
with carcinoma of the breast. The 99mTc sulfur colloid scan in this
patient, revealed metastatic liver disease. Gallium-67 demonstrated
no preferential affinity for the sites of metastases and is not
recommended in this organ evaluation. (A = anterior reclining,
UA = upright anterior, RL = right lateral, ANT = anterior whole body
67Ga rectilinear scan.)

References Chapter 2

1. Meissner, W.A., Warren, S. Sites of metastases at autopsy. In Pathology. Edited by W.A.D. Anderson, St. Louis, C.V. Mosby Co., 1: 538, 1971.

2. Brennan, M.J. Breast cancer. In Cancer Medicine. Edited by J.F. Holland and E. Frei. Philadephia, Lea and Febiger, p. 1785, 1973.

3. Nemoto, T., Dao, T.L. Significance of liver metastasis in women with disseminated breast cancer and undergoing endocrine ablative surgery. Cancer 19: 421, 1966.

4. Wagner, H.N., Jr., McAfee, J.G., Mozley, J.M. Diagnosis of liver disease by radioisotope scanning. Arch Intern Med 107: 324, 1961.

5. McAfee, J., Ause, R.G., Wagner, H.N. Diagnostic value of scintillation scanning of the liver. Arch Intern Med 116: 95, 1965.

6. Johnson, P.M. The Liver. In Clinical Scintillation Scanning. Freeman, L.M. and Johnson, P.M., eds. New York, Harper and Row, p. 260, 1969.

7. Mangum, J.F., Powell, M.R. Liver scintigraphy as an index of liver abnormality. J Nucl Med 14: 484, 1973.

8. Lunia, S., Parthasarathy, K.L., Bakshi, S., Bender, M.A. An evaluation of 99mTc-colloid liver scintiscans and their usefulness in metastatic workup: A review of 1,424 studies. J Nucl Med 16: 62, 1975.

9. Johnston, G.S., Jones, A.E. Sequential liver scanning. J Surg Oncol 1: 205, 1969.

10. Covington, E.E. Pitfalls in liver photoscans. Am J Roentgenol Radium Ther Nucl Med 109: 745, 1970.

11. Covington, E.E. The accuracy of liver photoscans. Am J Roentgenol Radium Ther Nucl Med 109: 742, 1970.

12. Conn, H.O., Spencer, R.P. Observer error in liver scan. Gastroenterology 62: 1085, 1972.

13. Poulose, K.P., Reba, R.C., Cameron, J.L., Wagner, H.N., Jr. The value and limitations of liver scanning for the detection of hepatic metastases in patients with cancer. J Indian Med Assoc 61: 199, 1973.

14. Jhingran, S.G., Jordan, L., Jahns, M.F., Haynie, T.P. Liver
     scintigrams compared with alkaline phosphatase and BSP
     determinations in the detection of metastatic carcinoma. J
     Nucl Med 12: 227, 1971.

15. Gollin, F.F., Sims, J. LeR., Cameron, J.R. Liver scanning and
     liver function tests. A comparative study. JAMA 187: 111,
     1964.

16. Castagna, J., Benfield, J.R., Yamada, H., Johnson, D.E.   The
     reliability of liver scans and function tests in detecting
     metastases. Surg Gynecol Obstet 134: 463, 1972.

17. Liewendahl, K., Schauman, K.O. Statistical evaluation of
     liver scanning in combination with liver function tests.
     Acta Med Scand 192: 395, 1972.

18. Poulose, K.P., Reba, R.C., DeLand, F.H., Wagner, H.N. Role of
     liver scanning in the preoperative evaluation of patients with
     cancer. Brit Med J 4: 585, 1969.

19. Davies, R.J., Vernon, M., Croft, D.N. Liver snaps and the
     detection of clinically unsuspected liver metastases. Lancet
     1: 279, 1974.

20. Hitzelberger, A.L., Parker, G.W., Durden, W.D., Johnston, G.S.
     Peritoneoscopy and radioisotope scintiscanning of the liver
     in the detection of hepatic metastases. Gastrointestinal
     Endoscopy, 13: 12, 1967.

21. Jones, A.E., Montgomery, J.L. Utility of combined hepatic
     scintigraphy and arteriography: Case examples of cirrhosis,
     hepastoma, and amebic abscess. J Surg Oncol 3: 657, 1971.

22. Freeman, L.M., Bernstein, R.G., Katz, M.C., Derman, A., Meng, C.
     Combined diagnostic approach of hepatic scanning and celiac
     angiography in the investigation of liver disease. J Nucl Med
     10: 628, 1969.

23. Swann, S.J., Boyce, C.L., Johnston, G.S., Jones, A.E.,
     Hardin, V. Patient positioning for hepatic scintigraphy.
     J Nucl Med Tech 1: 27, 1973.

24. Volpe, J.A., Morita, E.T., Johnston, G.S. The false positive
     technetium-99m hepatic scintiscan. J Surg Oncol 1: 345,
     1969.

25. Polcyn, R.E., Quinn, J.L., Gottschalk, A. Liver scan
     artifacts. J Nucl Med 9: 342, 1968.

26.   Milder, M.S., Larson, S.M., Swann, S.J. Johnston, G.S.
      False-positive liver scan due to breast prosthesis. J Nucl
      Med 14:   198, 1973.

27.   Bonte, F.J., Krohmer, J.S., Elmendorf, E., Presley, N.L.,
      Andrews, G.J., Scintillation scanning of the liver: II.
      Clinical applications. Amer J Roentgenol Radium Ther Nucl Med
      88:   275, 1962.

28.   Johnson, P.M. Sweeney, W.A.   False-positive hepatic scans
      J Nucl Med 8:   451, 1967.

29.   Richman, S.D., Ingle, J.N., Levenson, S.M., Tormey, D.C.,
      Jones, A.E., Johnston, G.S. The usefulness of gallium
      scintigraphy in primary and metastatic breast carcinoma. J
      Nucl Med 16:   560, 1975.

30.   Levenson, S.M., Ingle, J.N., Richman, S.D., Frankel, R.S.,
      Tormey, D.C., Jones, A.E., Johnston, G.S. Liver scanning in
      metastatic carcinoma of the breast. J Nucl Med 16:   545,
      1975.

31.   Mansfield, C.M., Kramer, S., Southard, M.E. The influence of
      treatment on the survival of patients with hepatic
      metastases diagnosed by liver scanning. Amer J Roentgenol
      Radium Ther Nucl Med 109:   749, 1970.

CHAPTER 3

Brain Scintigraphy

Alfred E. Jones, M.D.

Department of Nuclear Medicine
Clinical Center
National Institutes of Health
Bethesda, Maryland

Brain scintigraphy with 99mTc pertechnetate has been used for
evaluating patients with breast cancer at the time of the first
visit and for follow-up visits. This has proved to be of little
value in screening all patients with carcinoma of the breast for
possible brain metastases. Brain scanning is more properly applied
to the breast carcinoma patient who has neurologic signs or symptoms
(Chapter 1: Diagnostic Considerations in Breast Cancer).

The autopsy incidence of breast carcinoma metastatic to brain
varies from 10% (1) to 25% (2) and higher (3), while the autopsy
incidence of metastatic breast carcinoma involving the skeleton has
been reported as being 75% (12). The high incidence of skeletal
metastases is reflected by the frequent involvement of the calvarium
which in turn, can result in an abnormal 99mTc pertechnetate brain
scan (4,5). Thus it is important to determine whether the brain
scan abnormality is due to breast carcinoma metastatic to the skull
or to the brain or to both sites. This chapter attempts to provide
an integrated approach to the use of diphosphonate cranial images,
pertechnetate brain scans and 67Ga head views in the detection and
differentiation of cerebral breast carcinoma lesions from skull
metastases.

In 1967 a scintigraphic approach to separating metastatic
lesions of the brain from those of the skull was evaluated using
99mTc pertechnetate and the bone seeking material, ionic
strontium-87m. It was observed that 99mTc pertechnetate delineated
brain tumors and strontium-87m revealed bone tumors; thus it was
suggested that combined studies utilizing both radionuclides in the
same subject would be helpful in distinguishing brain tumors from

37

skull tumors (6). This same problem was more recently studied with
the newer bone seeking agent 99mTc diphosphonate, which was observed
to have a less specific localization within either primary or
metastatic neoplasms of the brain than did 99mTc pertechnetate (7).

Nevertheless 99mTc diphosphonate was found to localize in brain
lesions and to complicate the interpretation of bone scans of the
skull (8). It is known to accumulate in a variety of intracerebral
lesions such as cerebral infarction, chronic subdural hematoma,
arteriovenous malformation, inflammatory lesions and primary or
metastatic neoplasms. Thus while 99mTc pertechnetate has a better
tumor-to-brain ratio than 99mTc diphosphonate, the latter agent is
far superior in demonstrating metastases to the bony calvarium.
Considered in combination, the two scanning agents offer a potential
for differentiating breast carcinoma metastatic to the skull from
those metastases that are purely intracerebral.

A third agent with greater tumor specificity, such as 67Ga,
might prove helpful in cases where 99mTc pertechnetate and 99mTc
diphosphonate have provided inconclusive results (9).

As an aid to staging and planning of therapy, patients with
breast carcinoma were studied first with a liver scan, then a brain
scan, followed by a 99mTc diphosphonate rectilinear bone scan, and
finally a whole body rectilinear 67Ga scan. This routine proved
especially helpful in evaluating the calvarium and its contents for
metastatic breast carcinoma.

Immediately following the liver scan, the patient received 15mCi
of 99mTc pertechnetate along with 300 mg. of potassium perchlorate.
Thirty to 60 minutes later, a five view gamma camera brain study was
performed, collecting 300,000 counts per view.

Whole body bone scans were obtained two days after the 99mTc
pertechnetate brain scan, thereby providing enough time for a
reasonable clearance of the activity remaining from the brain study.
Since the rectilinear bone study provided only anterior and
posterior views of the head, additional lateral gamma camera views
of the skull and cervical spine were routinely obtained, collecting
50,000 counts per view. Immediately after completion of the bone
scan, 67Ga (50uCi/Kg body weight) was administered intravenously and
the patient returned 72 hours later for a whole body dual probe
rectilinear scan. Gallium-67 head views were not obtained unless
there was a suspicious area noted on the brain scan. Since it was
recognized that 67Ga was not particularly successful in detecting
metastatic breast carcinoma, whole body 67Ga scans were not required
of all patients during subsequent scintigraphic follow-up studies
(Chapter 1).

Of the N.I.H. patients who came to autopsy, 10 had proven brain
metastases. Three of these patients had lesions that were detected
by 99mTc pertechnetate brain scintigraphy. One of the three
patients had an abnormal 99mTc diphosphonate skull study. In
addition, two other patients had positive 99mTc diphosphonate skull
views only. Thus five of the 10 patients had abnormal views of the
brain or calvarium. Of the remaining five patients one had a lesion
in the posterior fossa, a difficult location to detect a lesion by
brain scan. The remaining four patients had normal brain and
calvarium scans within four weeks of autopsy. At autopsy two of
these patients had large lesions and there is no apparent reason why
they were not visible on brain scan. Two other patients had lesions
that were too small to be seen on brain scan.

The results of the 99mTc pertechnetate brain studies might have
been better if views were obtained later than 30 to 60 minutes after
dosing (10). This is evident in Fig. 3-1 where 99mTc pertechnetate
views at 30 minutes and 90 minutes are compared with 99mTc
diphosphonate and 67Ga views of a metastatic breast carcinoma lesion
within the brain. Skull views with 99mTc diphosphonate appear to be
best four hours after dosing (Fig. 3-2).

Routine 99mTc pertechnetate brain images may show no abnormality
in the presence of bony involvement of the calvarium. They should
be compared to the rectilinear 99mTc diphosphonate and 67Ga studies
and if possible with selected 99mTc diphosphonate gamma camera views
of the calvarium (Fig. 3-3). Routine lateral gamma camera views,
taken along with the 99mTc diphosphonate whole body rectilinear
study, are most productive in revealing and defining the extent of
metastatic breast carcinoma within the skull (Chapter 5, Figs. 5-6A
and B).

The correlation of brain scan abnormalities with metastases
within the calvarium is readily accomplished by comparing the brain
scan views with the 99mTc diphosphonate skull views and the skull
x-rays (Fig. 3-4). Progression of an abnormal 99mTc pertechnetate
study should also be compared with similar 99mTc diphosphonate views
and the skull films in order to more reliably credit the change in
brain scan to metastatic disease of the skull. Conversely,
successful therapy may be demonstrated by serial views of the skull
taken before and after therapy (Chapter 5, Fig. 5-5C).

When the bone scans and brain scans are positive in the same
area it is possible that contiguous meningeal spread may have
occurred since the close application of the dura to the calvarium
facilitates direct extension of the malignancy (11). In this group
of 10 patients with autopsy proven brain metastasis, two had
positive 99mTc diphosphonate skull views and meningeal metastases.
One of these two patients also had a left hemiparesis associated

with an abnormality on the right seen in the 99mTc pertechnetate brain scan. The diphosphonate image indicated diffuse disease throughout the calvarium in contrast to the 67Ga view which showed a localization within the abnormality detected in the pertechnetate brain scan (Fig. 3-6). The 67Ga appeared to detect the cerebral metastasis and differentiate the brain lesion from the diffuse metastases within the calvarium. Nevertheless, the localization of 67Ga may be no better than that of 99mTc diphosphonate or 99mTc pertechnetate within an intracerebral breast carcinoma metastasis (Fig. 3-1). The variable affinity of 67 Ga for intracerebral breast metastases appears to make it a worthwhile procedure to be employed when the 99mTc pertechnetate study is negative and there is a high suspicion of an intracerebral lesion. A negative 67Ga study offers no reassurance that an intracerebral lesion is not present.

In conclusion, routine 99mTc pertechnetate brain scintigraphy was not a satisfactory screening procedure in the detection of occult cerebral breast carcinoma metastases. Additional gamma camera head views were necessary for a thorough metastatic survey at the time of performing whole body 99mTc diphosphonate bone scans. When the 99mTc pertechnetate brain scan is negative or suspicious in a breast carcinoma patient with neurologic signs or symptoms, gamma camera head views with 99mTc diphosphonate and 67Ga may prove helpful.

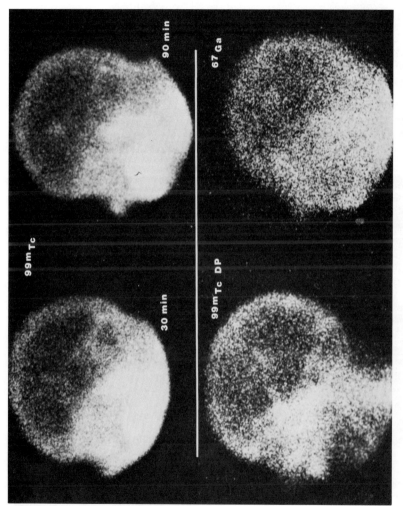

Fig. 3-1. Top: Left lateral images at 30 and 90 minutes following intravenous 99mTc pertechnetate. Note that this breast carcinoma lesion is seen more clearly at 90 minutes. Bottom: Left lateral 99mTc diphosphonate and 67Ga images of the same lesion as shown above. Both diphosphonate and 67Ga localized faintly in this lesion. This metastasis demonstrated a poor affinity for 67Ga in contrast to the lesion shown in Figs. 3-7 and 8.

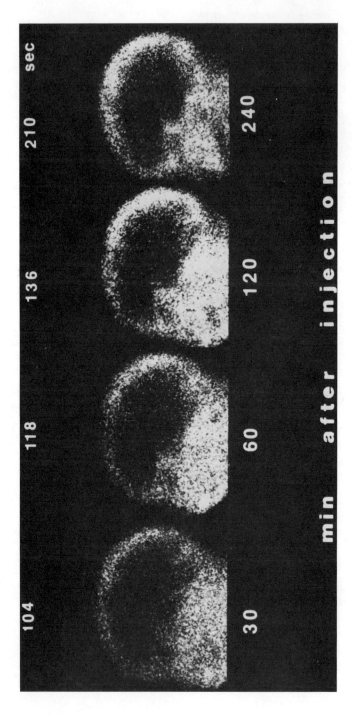

Fig. 3-2. The optimum time for collecting a 99mTc diphosphonate skull image was around 240 minutes after I.V. injection. Note the increasing length of time (seconds) required to collect the consecutive left lateral gamma camera images.

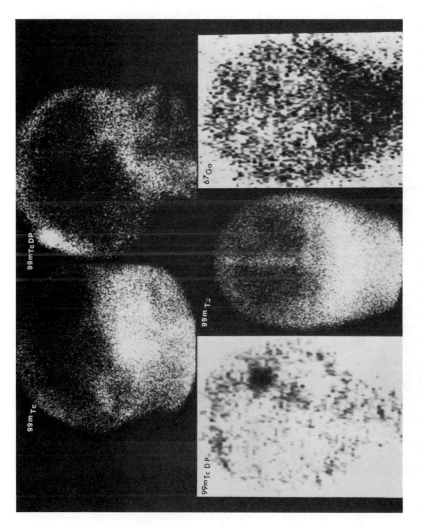

Fig. 3-3. Top: right lateral brain and skull images reveal an occipital lesion. A comparison of the 99mTc pertechnetate brain images with selected 99mTc diphosphonate gamma camera skull views will frequently provide further clarification of the rectilinear images. Bottom: from left to right, posterior rectilinear skull, posterior camera brain, and a posterior rectilinear 67Ga head view of the same patient seen in the top row.

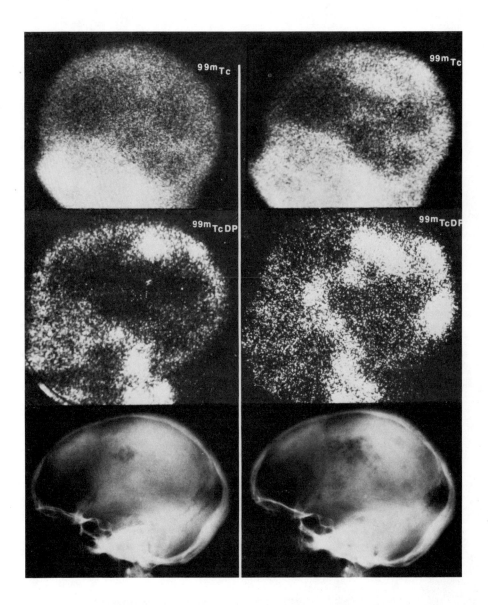

Fig. 3-4. Top: 99mTc pertechnetate brain scans; middle: 99mTc
diphosphonate skull views; bottom: lateral skull x-rays. All views
on the right were obtained 12 months following those on the left.
The abnormalities seen on brain scan were clarified by the bone scan
and lateral skull x-rays. Serial studies show the progress of the
metastases. The 99mTc diphosphonate skull views defined
the full extent of the lesions that are seen on the skull x-rays.

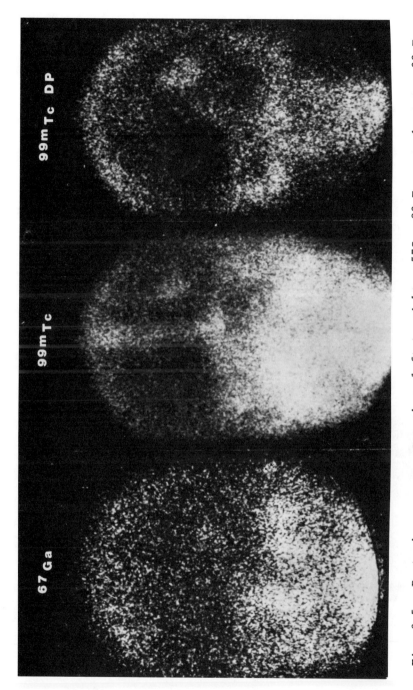

Fig. 3-5. Posterior gamma camera views left to right: 57Ga, 99mTc pertechnetate; 99mTc diphosphonate. The bony lesion was visualized in all three studies but most clearly with 99mTc diphosphonate. (Compare with Figs. 3-1 and 7 which show intracerebral breast carcinoma metastases).

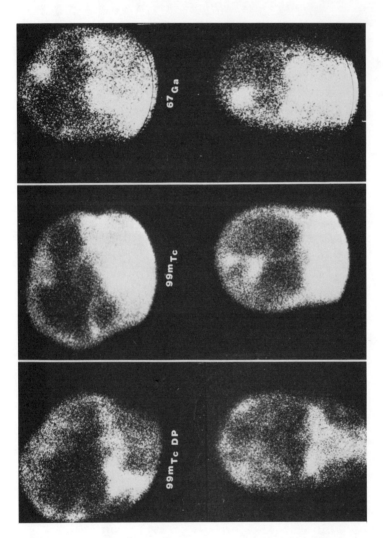

Fig. 3-6. Comparative right lateral (top) and anterior (bottom) gamma camera views of metastatic breast carcinoma. Note the extensive bony involvement seen with diphosphonate. The 67Ga selectively localized within an area suggesting a discrete tumoral component located within the defect seen on the pertechnetate brain images. The patient was known to have an extension of breast carcinoma involving the right cerebral hemisphere with a resulting left hemiparesis.

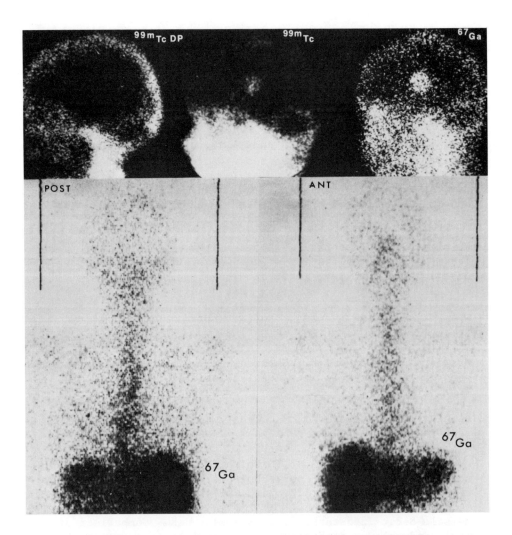

Fig. 3-7: Top row: An intracerebral breast carcinoma metastasis
was clearly seen on both the 99mTc pertechnetate and 67Ga gamma
camera views but was not visible with 99mTc diphosphonate. As seen
in Fig. 3-6, the soft tissue tumoral component is clearly visible
with 67Ga as opposed to lesions of the bony calvarium which are
poorly detected with 67Ga (Fig. 3-5) Bottom: The same lesion is
inadequately visualized in the posterior (left) and anterior (right)
rectilinear images.

References Chapter 3

1. Brennan, M.J. Breast Cancer. In Cancer Medicine. Edited by
    J.F. Holland and E. Frei III, Philadelphia, Lea and Febiger
    p. 1769, 1973.

2. Viadana, E., Bross, I.D.J., Pickren, J.W. An autopsy study
    of some routes of dissemination of cancer of the breast. Br J
    Cancer 27: 336, 1973.

3. Abrams, H.L., Spiro, R., Goldstein, N. Metastases in carcinoma.
    Analysis of 1000 autopsied cases. Cancer 3: 74, 1950.

4. Haynie, T.P., III, Radionuclide imaging of brain, liver and
    bone in disseminated breast cancer. In Breast Cancer - Early and
    Late. Chicago, Yearbook Medical Publishers, p. 301, 1970.

5. Whitley, J.E., Witcofski, R.L., Bolliger, T.T., Maynard, C.D.
    Tc99m in the visualization of neoplasms outside the brain.
    Amer J Roent 96: 706, 1966.

6. Tow, D.E., Wagner, H.N., Jr. Scanning for tumors of brain and
    bone: comparison of sodium pertechnetate Tc99m and ionic
    strontium 87m. JAMA 199: 610, 1967.

7. Grames, G.M., Jansen, C., Carlsen, E.N., Davidson, T.R. The
    abnormal bone scan in intracranial lesions. Radiol
    115: 129, 1975.

8. Maynard, C.D., Hanner, T.G., Witcofski, R.L. Positive brain
    scans due to lesions of the skull. Arch Neurol 18: 93, 1968.

9. Jones, A.E., Frankel, R.S., DiChiro, G., Johnston, G.S. Brain
    scintigraphy with 99mTc pertechnetate, 99mTc polyphosphate and
    67Ga Citrate. Radiol 112: 123, 1974.

10. Meisel, S-B., Izenstark, J.L., Siemsen, J.K. Comparison of
    early and delayed technetium and mercury brain scanning.
    Radiol 109: 117, 1973.

11. Russell, D.S., Rubinstein, L.J., Lunsden, C.E. Pathology
    of Tumors of The Nervous System. Baltimore, The Williams and
    Wilkens Co., p. 225, 1963.

CHAPTER 4

Breast Scintigraphy

Steven D. Richman, M.D.

Department of Nuclear Medicine
National Institutes of Health
Bethesda, Maryland

Conventional film mammography and xeroradiography are the
fundamental and most widely used techniques for the study of breast
disease. Thermography is becoming established as a sensitive
preliminary screening method capable of detecting early breast
carcinoma. Thorough investigation with these modalities, in
conjunction with clinical examination, yields greater than 90%
diagnostic accuracy. Yet, equivocal cases occur all too frequently,
especially in the young glandular breast. A complementary,
non-invasive technique for the early detection of breast carcinoma
differentiation of benign and malignant lesions has become a
continuing goal in nuclear medicine.

Early attempts at isotopic breast tumor detection were
relatively unrewarding. Mammary scintigraphy was initially proposed
utilizing surface measurements of 32P (1) and 42K (2). Mercurial
compounds have been actively studied as breast tumor scanning
agents. In 1965, Sodee (3) demonstrated 197Hg-chlormerodrin
localization in two of three breast carcinomas using a rectilinear
scanner. Buchwald (4), using 197HgCl2, studied 26 patients with
this malignancy of whom 18 were positive and four were questionable.
Sannazzari (5) reported nine of ten breast carcinomas visualized by
rectilinear scan using 197HgCl2. The high absorbed radiation dose
to the kidneys with these compounds has limited their clinical
application. Bonte using 131I-human serum albumin had difficulty
with rectilinear image quality, as demonstrated by two fair and two
poor scans in patients with large primary breast carcinomas.

The neoplastic localization of 67 Ga-citrate (67Ga) has
undergone intensive clinical investigation. The affinity for 67Ga

varies with the origin of the neoplasm. Primary breast carcinoma has proved less detectable than lymphoma or lung carcinoma (7)(8). Most studies, utilizing rectilinear scans, have reported suboptimal 50 to 60% detection rates for breast carcinoma.

The radiopharmaceutical most suitable for such scintigraphic study, 99mTc pertechnetate, was first proposed for extracranial tumor localization by Witley in 1966 (9). A positive finding occurred in the single breast carcinoma investigated. Cancroft (10) applied gamma camera techniques to demonstrate focal accumulation in four patients with breast carcinoma. There was no abnormal accumulation in two patients with benign breast disease. Villarreal (11) subsequently evaluated six patients with breast carcinoma demonstrating tumor localization of 99mTc pertechnetate in five. Of 30 cases with benign breast disease, six demonstrated "false positive" localization of 99mTc pertechnetate.

In a study to evaluate and compare the usefulness of 99mTc pertechnetate and 67Ga for radionuclide breast scintigraphy (12), lateral, medial and cranio-caudal gamma camera breast views were performed 15-60 minutes following the intravenous injection of 10-15 millicuries of 99mTc pertechnetate. The patient was placed in the sitting or erect position and was drapped with a lead apron to allow only the breast in question to be exposed for scintigraphic study (Fig. 4-1 A,B,C). Cobalt-57 markers are placed on the collimator to note the nipple and axilla. The high resolution, low energy collimator was used for lateral and medial views; 300,000 counts were obtained with an approximate time of 200 seconds for each view. The cranio-caudal view with positioning similar to conventional mammography utilizes the pinhole collimator with a 4.5 millimeter tungsten insert. Satisafctory images are obtained in 250 seconds with 50-80 thousand counts.

Gallium-67 (50uCi/Kg of body weight) breast scans were obtained 48 hours after intravenous administration. Lateral and medial views were identical in positioning and shielding with those of 99mTc pertechnetate breast scintigraphy. The high energy collimator was used to accumulate 50,000 counts per view in approximately 300 seconds. The count rate has proved inadequate for cranio-caudal 67Ga gamma camera breast imaging.

Sixteen cases of breast carcinoma have been evaluated with 14 demonstrating abnormal 99mTc accumulation (Table 1). Discrete, focal concentration of 99m was the most common finding. There was excellent anatomical correlation with clinical, radiographic and histologic localization of breast malignancies. Of 10 patients with proven breast carcinoma, five had positive 67Ga scans, but five failed to demonstrate abnormal concentration. When both radionuclide scintiscans were positive, lesions were better visualized with 99mTc pertechnetate. Of 17 patients

Table I

Scintigraphic Mammography
In Breast Carcinoma

	Positive	Negative	Accuracy
99mTcO$_4$	14	2	14/16 = 88 %
67Ga	5	5	5/10 = 50 %

Table II

Scintigraphic Mammography In
Benign Breast Disease

	Positive	Negative	Accuracy
99mTcO$_4$	5	12	12/17 = 70 %
67Ga	1	9	9/10 = 90 %

with biopsy proven benign breast disease, five had abnormal localization of 99mTc pertechnetate (Table II). Gallium-67 demonstrated one false positive in 10 cases of proven benign breast disease.

Caution is necessary in supporting the validity of 99mTc pertechnetate breast scintigraphy. The high "false-positive" rate limits the use of 99mTc pertechnetate breast scintigraphy for differential diagnosis and for screening purposes. The excellent correlation between malignancy and positive breast scintigraphy (88%) may prove useful in the preoperative documentation of the extent of disease or in the evaluation of the response to therapy. Gallium-67 scintigraphy, though, a useful corroborative study when positive, is an insensitive agent for the detection of breast carcinoma. Our attempts at gamma camera scintigraphy have not improved the diagnostic accuracy noted with rectilinear scanning.

Limitations of specificity similar to that encountered with 99mTc pertechnetate have been reported with bone imaging agents employed for tumor scanning. Berg (13) reported the incidental finding of increased 99mTc-diphosphonate uptake in primary breast carcinoma in two patients undergoing skeletal rectilinear scans. Serafini (14) obtained gamma camera images demonstrating focal accumulation of 99mTc-diphosphonate or 99mTc-polyphosphate in 82% of 17 patients with breast carcinoma. However, 36% of patients with benign breast disease had positive scans as well.

Successful breast scintigraphy for tumor detection requires more selective radionuclides than those presently available. However, because of its low radiation dose and its non-invasiveness, the concept merits further investigation.

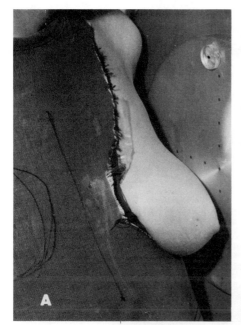
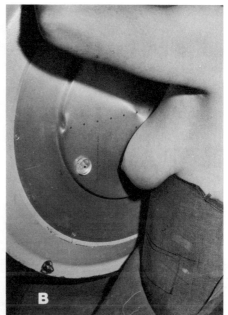
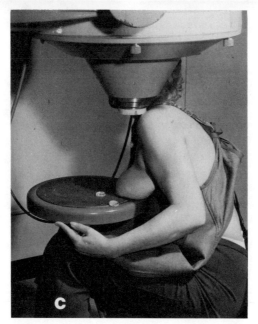

Fig. 4-1. The patient is positioned for lateral (A), medial
(B), and cranio-caudal (C) gamma camera breast scintigraphy.

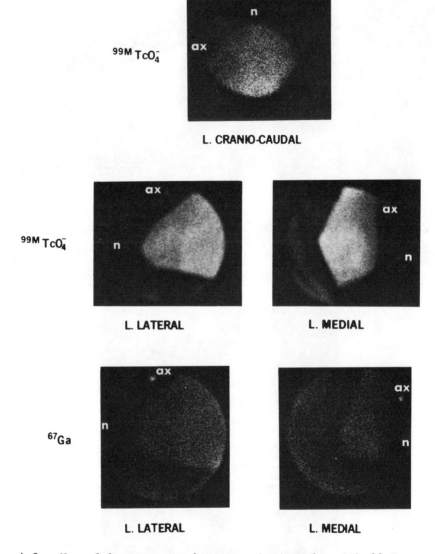

Fig. 4-2.   Normal homogeneous breast scintigraphy with 99mTc
pertechnetate and 67Ga citrate.   There is a relative increase in
radionuclide accumulation close to the chest wall in all views.   The
sharp delineation in the medial views is caused by the lead
shielding against the chest wall.   (n = nipple, ax = axilla
in all of the following illustrations).

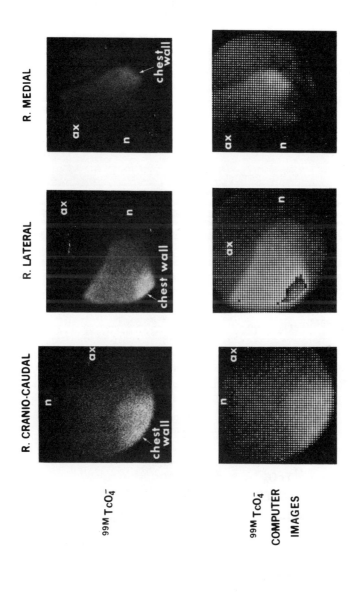

Fig. 4-3. The normal breast silhouette in 99mTc pertechnetate cranio-caudal, lateral and medial breast scintigraphy. Respective computer images are shown.

R. CRANIO-CAUDAL

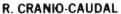

MAMMOGRAM

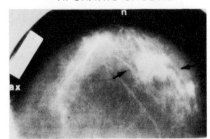

XERORADIOGRAPH

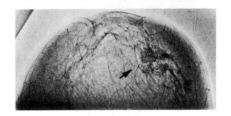

$^{99M}TcO_4^-$
SCINTIPHOTO

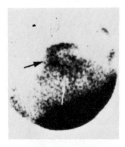

$^{99M}TcO_4^-$
COMPUTER
IMAGE

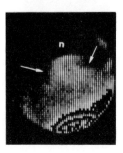

Fig. 4-4A. Cranio-caudal mammogram, xeroradiograph and 99mTc
pertechnetate breast scan demonstrate a malignant mass with good
anatomic correlation.

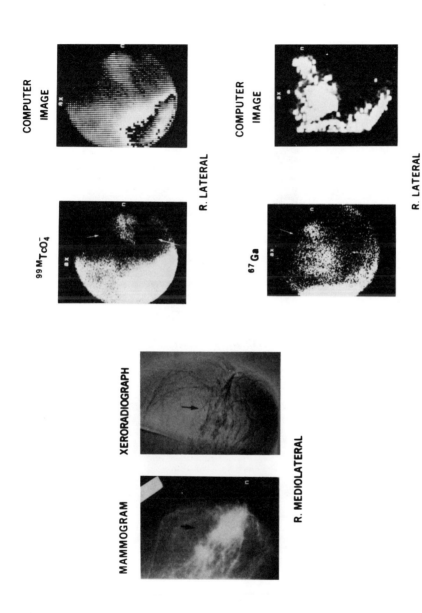

Fig. 4-4B. In the same patient, corresponding mediolateral roentgenographic studies and lateral radionuclide scintiscans show breast cancer. Computer representations can be used to confirm the abnormality.

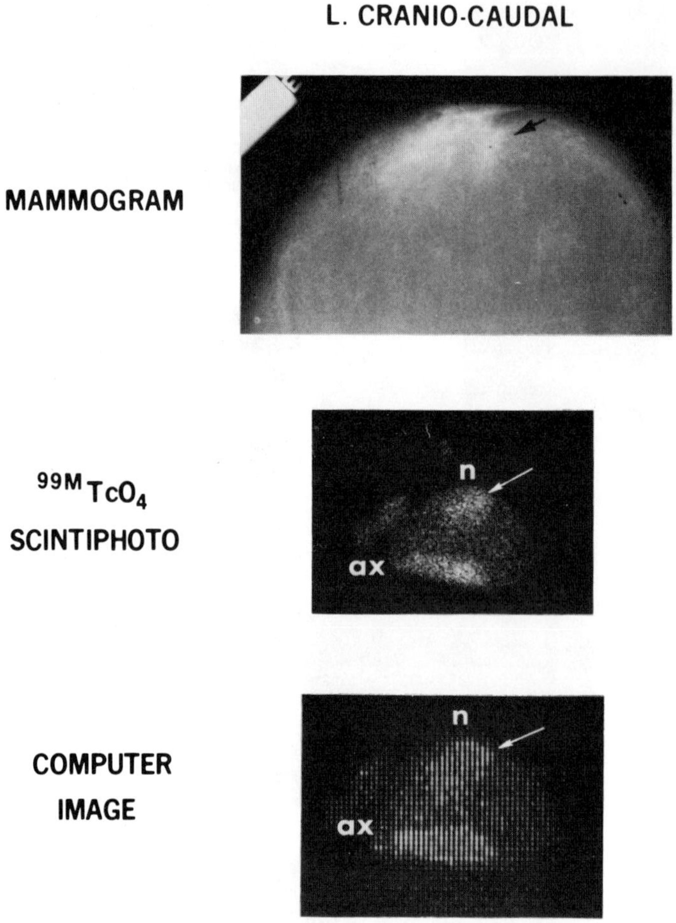
L. CRANIO-CAUDAL
MAMMOGRAM
99M TcO4
SCINTIPHOTO
n
ax
COMPUTER
IMAGE
n
ax

Fig. 4-5A. Cranio-caudal roentgenograph and scintiscan reveal sub-areolar breast carcinoma.

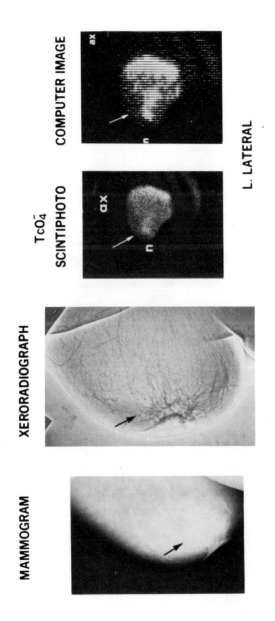

Fig. 4-5B. Mediolateral mammogram and xeroradiograph, and lateral breast scan demonstrate the same tumor. The computer image reveals a larger abnormality than previously suspected by all other means. This was confirmed at surgery.

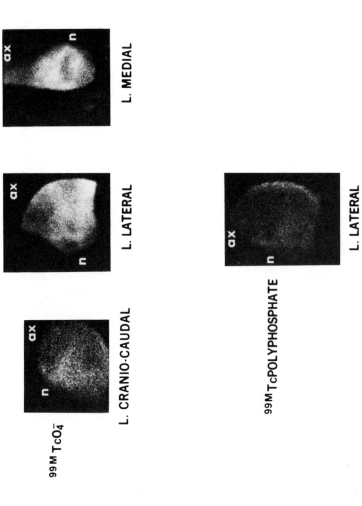

Fig. 4-6. Mottled, irregular, increased uptake of 99mTc pertechnetate followed a recent aspiration biopsy in this 48 year old woman with breast carcinoma. 99mTc polyphosphate also localized in this soft tissue tumor.

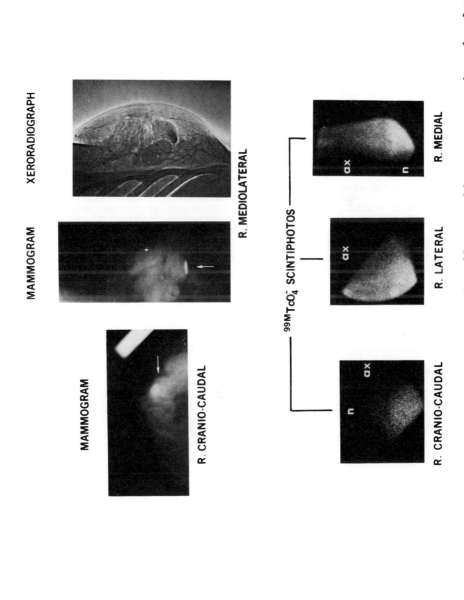

Fig. 4-7. Clinical breast evaluation in this 43 year old woman was equivocal. Large cysts with "milk of calcium" in several cysts were noted in the mammogram. Breast scintigraphy with 99mTc pertechnetate was negative and biopsy was benign.

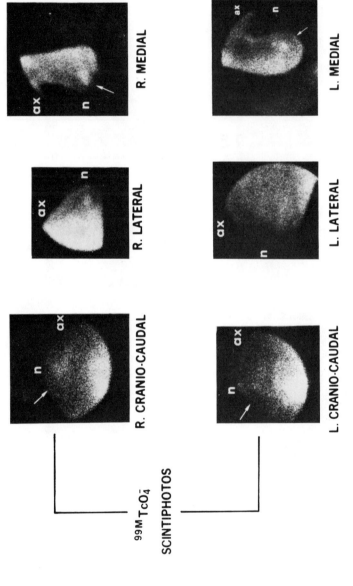

Fig. 4-8. Bilateral focal breast accumulations of 99mTc pertechnetate were noted in this patient. Abnormalities are best seen in the medial views. The left was carcinoma and a mastectomy was performed. Biopsy of the right breast demonstrated only fibrocystic disease.

References Chapter 4

1. Low-Beer, B.V.A., Bell, H.G., McCorkle, H.J. Measurement of radioactive phosphorus in breast tumors in situ: A possible diagnostic procedure; preliminary report. Radiology 47: 492, 1946.

2. Baker, H.W., Nathanson, I.T., Selverstone, B. Use of radioactive potassium (K42) in the study of benign and malignant breast tumors. New Eng J Med 252: 612, 1955.

3. Sodee, B.D., Renner, R.R., Di Stefano, B. Photoscanning localization of tumor, utilizing chlormerodrin mercury-197. Radiology 84: 873, 1965.

4. Buchwald, W., Diethelm, L., Wolf, R. Scintigraphic delineation of carcinoma of the breast and parasternal lymph nodes. In Radioactive Isotopes in the Localization of Tumors. Edited by V.R. McCready. New York, Grune and Stratton, p. 138, 1969.

5. Sanazzari, G.L., Comino, E., Negri, G.L., Baracchi, G. Radiographic and scintigraphic study of normal and pathologic breast. Minerva Med 63: 1532, 1972.

6. Bonte, F.J., Curry, T.S. III, Oelze, R.E., Greenberg, A.J. Radioisotope scanning of tumors. Am J Roentgenol Radium Ther Nucl Med 100: 801, 1967.

7. Hayes, R.L., Edwards, C.L. New applications of tumor localizing radiopharmaceuticals. IAEA Symposium on Medical Radioisotope Scintigraphy. IAEA, Vienna, 2: 531, 1973.

8. Edwards, C.L., Hayes, R.L. Localization of tumors with radioisotopes. In Clinical Uses of Radionuclides: Critical Comparison with Other Techniques. Oak Ridge, Tennessee, p. 618, 1971.

9. Whitley, J.E., Witcofski, R.L., Bolliger, T.T., Maynard, C.D. 99mTc in the visualization of neoplasms outside the brain. Am J Roentgenol Radium Ther Nucl Med 96: 706, 1966.

10. Cancroft, E.T., Goldsmith, S.J. 99mTc pertechnetate scintigraphy as an aid in the diagnosis of breast masses. Radiology 106: 441, 1973.

11. Villarreal, R.L., Parkey, R.W., Bonte, F.J. Experimental pertechnetate mammography. Radiology 111: 657, 1974.

12.   Richman, S.D., Brodey, P.A., Frankel, R.S., De Moss, E.V.,
      Tormey D.C., Johnston, G.S.   Breast scintigraphy
      99mTc pertechnetate and 67Ga citrate.   J Nucl Med
      16:   293, 1975.

13.   Berg, G.R., Kalisher, L., Osmond, J.D., Pendergrass, H.P.,
      Potsaid, M.S.   99mTc diphosphonate concentration in primary
      breast carcinoma.   Radiology 109:   393, 1973.

14.   Serafini, A. M., Raskin, M.M., Zand, L.C., Watson, D.D.
      Radionuclide breast scanning in carcinoma of the breast.   J Nuc
      Med 15:   1149, 1974.

CHAPTER 5

Skeletal Scintigraphy

Robert S. Frankel, M.D.
Stanley M. Levenson, M.D.

Department of Nuclear Medicine
National Institutes of Health
Bethesda, Maryland

Since the advent of instrumentation capable of recording images
of the whole body, bone scintigraphy has assumed an increasingly
important role in the detection of primary and secondary bone
lesions. With the recent introduction of various 99mTc phosphate
bone seeking radionuclides, resultant improvement in image quality
and scanning accuracy has added even more importance to this
procedure in the investigation of suspected metastatic bone disease
(1-5).

It is commonly felt that a metastatic bone lesion must be 50 to
70 percent demineralized before becoming visible on roentgenogram
(6,7). Since localization of bone seeking radionuclides is
dependent on bone turnover and regional blood flow, rather than
demineralization, it is possible to detect the presence of
metastases at an earlier stage than with radiographs. Numerous
reports document the consistent superiority of bone scans over
radiographs and clinical evidence of pain for the detection of early
metastatic skeletal lesions (5-14). Charkes et al. reported 12
patients with various neoplasms in which the roentgenogram was
normal and strontium-85 bone scan abnormal; biopsy or autopsy
specimens from eight (67%) confirmed metastatic tumor (14). Hopkins and
Kristensen correlated roentgenograms of the axial skeleton, skull
and extremities with fluorine-18 and 99mTc polyphosphate bone scans
in 79 patients (13). Thirty patients (38%) demonstrated lesions on
the scan which were not detected roentgenographically. Metastases
were confirmed by subsequent x-ray changes, biopsy, autopsy or
relief of bone pain after radiotherapy. Twenty (67%) of these
patients were asymptomatic.

In the National Institutes of Health breast cancer population, approximately 96% of documented or highly suspected metastatic bone lesions were present on the bone scan. Less than 3% of the metastatic bone lesions were initially detected by radiograph with a normal scan, whereas 30% of the lesions were initially detected by scan alone (15). This data is in keeping with most previously published reports (5,8,10,11).

Sklaroff and Charkes suggest that bone scans may also be of value in the early postoperative period if not performed preoperatively (11). Using strontium-85, 10 of 64 patients (15%) were found to have abnormal scans and normal roentgenograms shortly after radical mastectomy. The stage of disease at mastectomy was not defined, however all patients had "significant" preoperative adenopathy and histologically positive ipsilateral axillary lymph nodes.

Hoffman and Marty studied 47 patients with pathologic Stage I or II breast cancer within three months of radical mastectomy; 19 (40%) had abnormal strontium-87m bone scans (12). Sixteen subsequently demonstrated skeletal metastases either by biopsy, autopsy or roentgenographic changes. Roentgenograms and bone scans were compared in seven Stage I patients. Both modalities revealed abnormalities in two patients, while three patients had completely normal studies. One patient had a positive scan and negative roentgenograms, and one patient had positive roentgenograms and a negative scan. Of 18 Stage II patients, two were abnormal by both modalities, 10 were normal, and six demonstrated positive scans with negative roentgenograms.

The importance of including the bone scan in the initial diagnostic evaluation of a patient with a breast mass either suspicious for or proven as cancer, has been elaborated upon in Chapter 1. The presence of unsuspected skeletal metastases has a definite bearing on the mode of therapy (12).

Although a significant percentage of lesions are not initially present on the radiographs when detected by scan, the majority of these do appear radiographically within 2-6 months (Fig. 5-3A,B,C,). Once present on bone roentgenogram, serial radiographs are a useful way of following progression of the lesion since its size and response to therapy can be evaluated. Serial bone scans have not been particularly helpful in evaluating the activity of a lesion. In the presence of persistently abnormal skeletal scintigraphs, radiographs often reveal sclerosis in the healing stage. Although this often cannot be differentiated from sclerosis in an active osteoblastic metastasis, the changing radiographic pattern appears more useful.

The procedure of whole body bone scintigraphy consists of the intravenous administration of 10 mCi of 99mTc diphosphonate with the site of injection being recorded to avoid later misinterpretation. A three to four hour waiting period is then allowed for clearance of 99mTc diphosphonate from the soft tissues. The patient is requested to void prior to the scanning procedure in order to optimize visualization of pelvic structures.

Since those referred for whole body bone imaging had been recently studied with brain and liver scintigraphy, adequate time was allowed for the residual tracer activity to decay and clear from the patient. It was most desirable to allow a period of 48 hours to elapse. When skeletal imaging was performed first, brain and liver scintigraphy were performed the following day.

Whole body bone images were obtained with a 5 inch dual probe rectilinear scanner capable of producing 5:1 reduction images. The patient was placed in a supine position with arms and legs closely adducted and fully extended. The head was placed with the face directed upward. Following the whole body bone scan, a gamma camera view of the cervical spine was obtained with the patient's body facing into the camera and head turned sideways. All patients received right and left lateral gamma camera head views which frequently detected metastases to the cranial vault, that were either unclear or not seen on the rectilinear scans. Bilateral rectilinear cranial views, obtained as part of the whole skeletal scan, were significantly inferior to multiple gamma camera scintiphotos. This may be partially due to the patient's difficulty in maintaining a direct lateral position on the scanning table. At present however, the camera is considered the instrument of choice for cranial vault imaging. Further "spot" gamma camera views were obtained to examine other suspicious areas seen on rectilinear scan and to evaluate symptomatic regions.

Several potential pitfalls of bone scan interpretation in patients with breast carcinoma must be kept in mind. These include: contamination of clothing by urine, tracer extravation at the injection site and a contaminated alcohol sponge retained by the patient. Camera views will usually clarify these artefacts. Since benign lesions also appear as areas of increased uptake on the scan, these too must be distinguished from metastatic disease. Therefore, it is always necessary to consider the possibility of a recent fracture, benign bone tumor or Paget's disease (Fig. 5-18), before ascribing an abnormal radionuclide accumulation to metastatic disease. If such benign lesions can be reasonably ruled out by history, physical and radiographic evaluations, the accuracy of an abnormal bone scan as an indication of metastasis approaches 95%.

Soft tissue localization of bone seeking radionuclides must be recognized as such and not interpreted as skeletal in origin. Localization in the region of a recent mastectomy site can usually be differentiated from rib lesions by its diffuse rather than discrete nature of appearance (Fig. 5-11A). Accumulation of 99mTc diphosphonate has also been seen in a cancerous breast prior to its removal (Fig. 5-17), as well as in normal breast tissue. Asymmetries of 99mTc diphosphonate localization are frequently noted following mastectomy and radiation therapy; respectively, these demonstrate diffuse, unilateral thoracic increases and decreases in radioactivity (Fig. 5-6A). In other areas that have received radio-therapy, diminished 99mTc diphosphonate activity may also be noted.

Radionuclide accumulation in the skull can present interpretive difficulties since 99mTc phosphate compounds accumulate in cerebral metastases or cerebral infarcts, as well as in cranial vault metastases (17). Localization of 99mTc diphosphonate in brain lesions is often less intense and more diffuse than when it is seen in metastases to the skull (Chapter 3 Fig. 3-1 and 5).

On occasion, a patient with diffuse skeletal metastases may present with a normal appearing bone scan (5,18,19). These cases have been unusual in their clarity of bony definition. The ribs are particularly well delineated. Although there is an increased amount of radioactivity in the skeleton, the lack of asymmetries lead the viewer to falsely believe that the scan is normal (Fig. 5-15A).

Following chemotherapy, bone scan abnormalities may show an increased amount of radioactivity, or new areas may appear. These can be misconstrued as progression of disease when in fact, healing with increased osteoblastic activity is the explanation. In this situation, the differentiation of disease progression from regression is aided by knowledge of the patient's clinical status.

Since the labeled phosphate bone imaging agents are cleared by the kidneys, it is of value to observe the position, size, and intensity of renal radionuclide localization. When a significant renal asymmetry is noted, there is an 85% chance of some renal abnormality (20,21). Ureteral visualization and bladder contour should also be considered.

In summary, whole body bone scans provide information concerning the site and extent of disease in patients with primary and metastatic carcinoma. The procedure may be repeated during and following therapy in order to assess the response to treatment or to detect recurrent sites of disease. Whole body bone scintigraphy has proven an invaluable aid in the investigation of breast carcinoma metastatic to bone. Its superiority to radiographic studies in the detection of early metastatic bone lesions is well documented. As

with other nuclear medical procedures, it should not be used in an
isolated manner, but rather as an adjunct to other available
modalities.

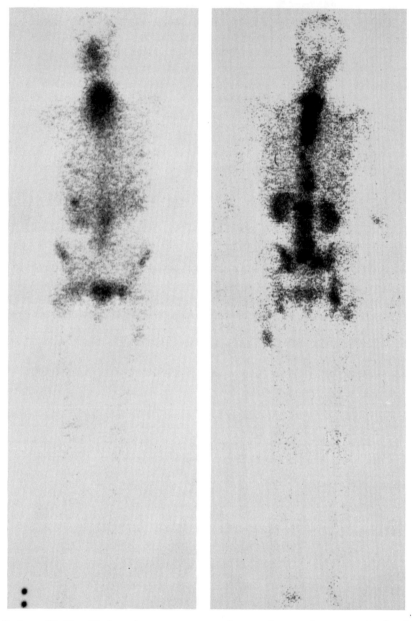

Fig. 5-1. 99mTc diphosphonate scans (anterior and posterior) show
diffuse metastases evidenced by multiple areas of increased nuclide
concentration in the anterior ribs, spine, sacrum, left sacroiliac
joint, right ischium, right femoral head, and proximal third of the
left femoral shaft. The intensity of uptake in the upper thoracic
spine is so great that activity is seen to "shine through" on the
anterior view. Radiographs also showed diffuse skeletal metastases.

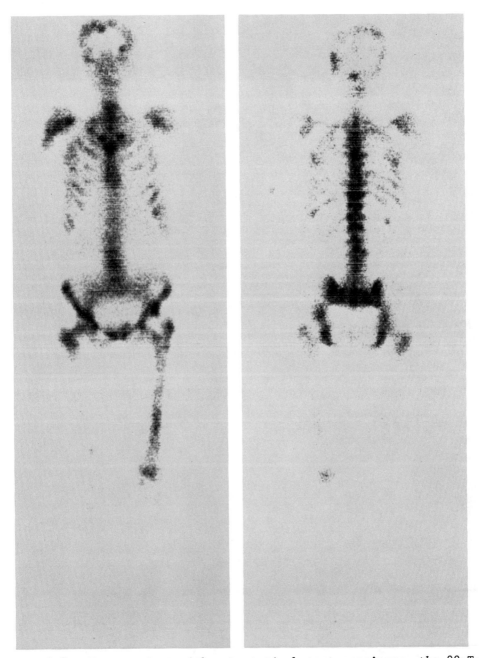

Fig. 5-2. In a patient with metastatic breast carcinoma, the 99mTc
diphosphonate scans show abnormal nuclide accumulation in the skull,
both shoulders, ribs, entire spine, pelvis and left femur.
Radiographic skeletal survey was also abnormal but did not detect as
many of the skull and rib lesions.

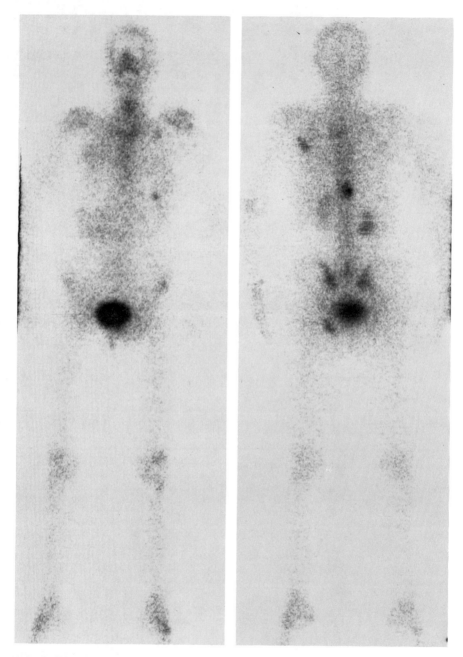

Fig. 5-3A. Anterior and posterior whole body scans with 99mTc diphosphonate show areas of increased uptake in the left anterior rib cage, left posterior rib cage or scapular tip, lower thoracic spine, lower lumbar spine, scaroiliac joints, and left ischium.

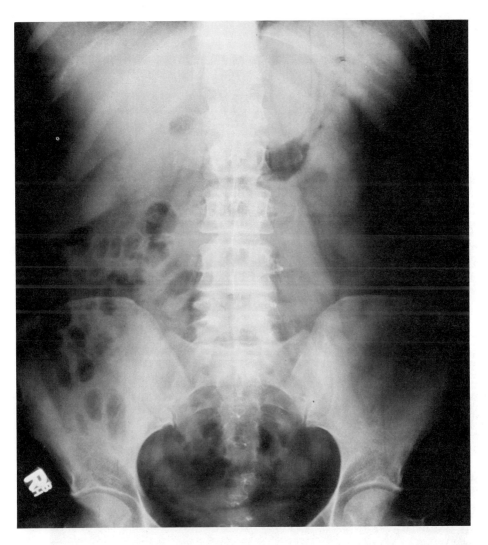

Fig. 5-3B. The only apparent metastatic lesion on the radiographic survey of this patient was in the left ischium. All other areas either became abnormal on radiographs within the ensuing nine months or became clinically symptomatic.

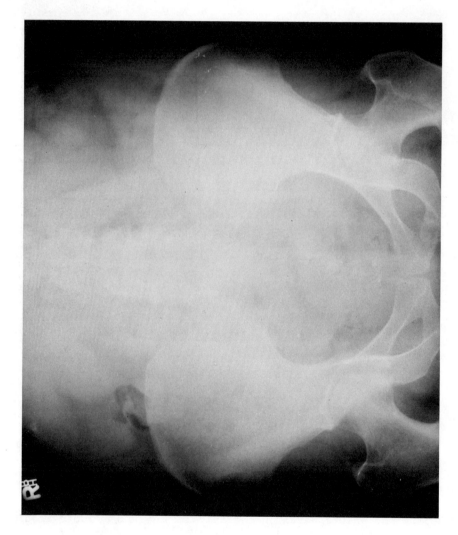

Fig. 5-3C. See caption of Fig. 5-3B.

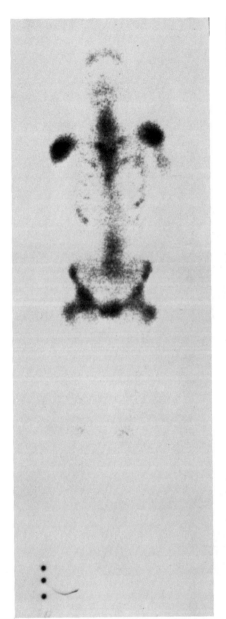
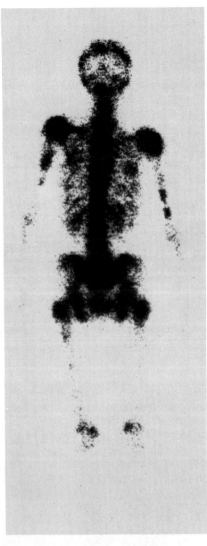

Fig. 5-4A. 99mTc diphosphonate scans on this patient with bilateral
shoulder pain reveal increased nuclide accumulations in the
shoulders and humeral shafts bilaterally. There is also diffusely
increased uptake in the spine suggestive of diffuse metastatic
involvement. Uptake throughout the pelvis is greater than normal,
especially in the ischii and femoral heads bilaterally and the
proximal portion of the left femoral shaft on the posterior scan.

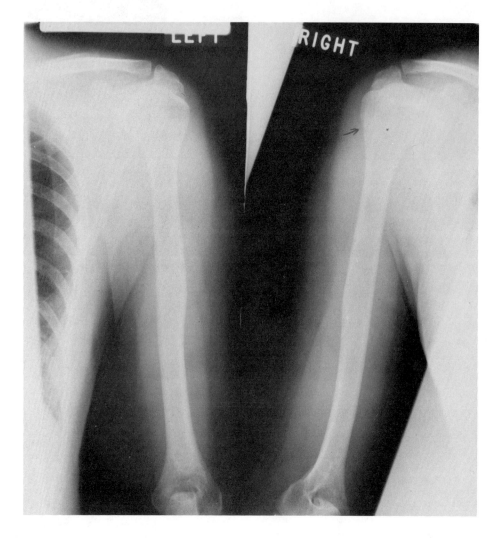

Fig. 5-4B. Radiographs of the shoulders and humeri show only
minimal erosive changes in the right upper humeral shaft. Films two
months later continued to be normal except for this one finding.

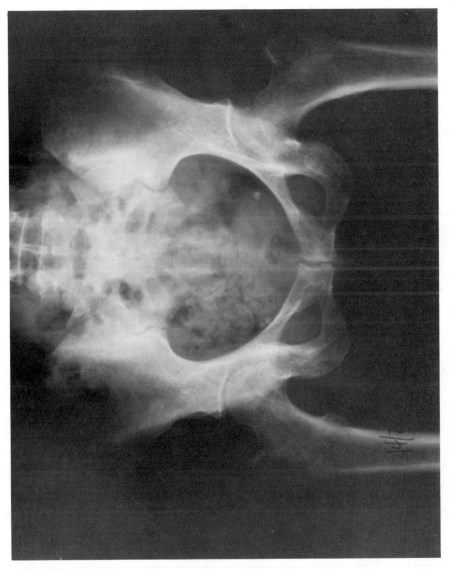

Fig. 5-4C. Radiography of the pelvis shows no definite abnormalities. Two months later, the patient developed diffuse pelvic pain with a persistent normal radiograph.

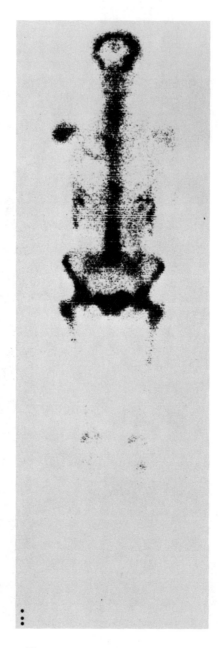

Fig. 5-5A. Anterior 99mTc diphosphonate bone image of this patient
shows multiple metastatic sites including the skull, right shoulder,
thoraco-lumbar spine, ribs, and much of the pelvis.

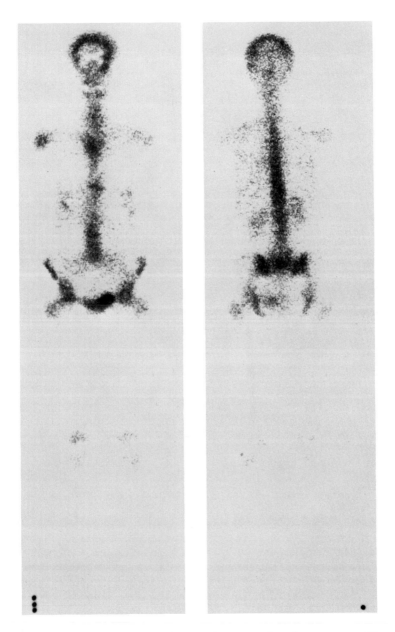

Fig. 5-5B. A follow-up anterior and posterior bone scan five months later, post-therapy, shows significant improvement. Note decreased localization of bone agent in the anterior chest bilaterally. This occurred following radiation therapy to these areas.

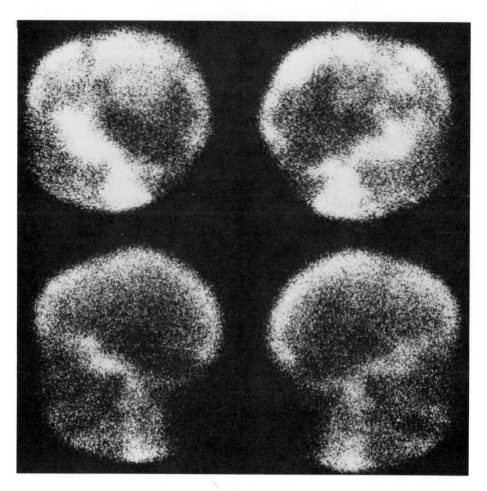

Fig. 5-5C. The usefulness of skeletal imaging in following the
course of the metastatic lesions as well as the superiority of
camera images over rectilinear views for skull lesions is evident in
this case. Left and right lateral skull views above, were obtained
prior to therapy; those below, following therapy.

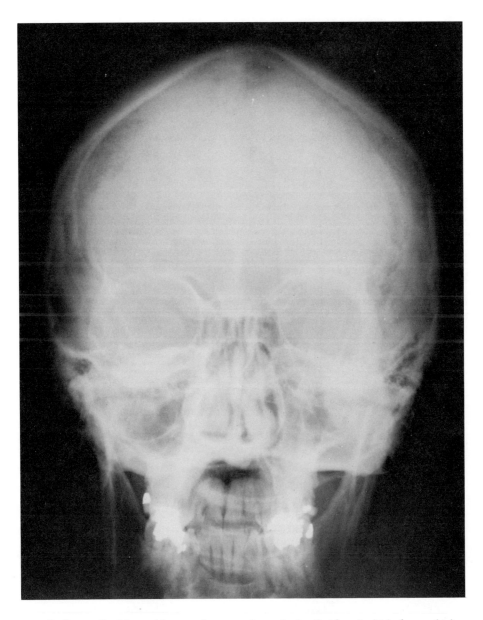

Fig. 5-5D. Skull radiographs at the time of the initial positive
scan of the head, were interpreted as normal.

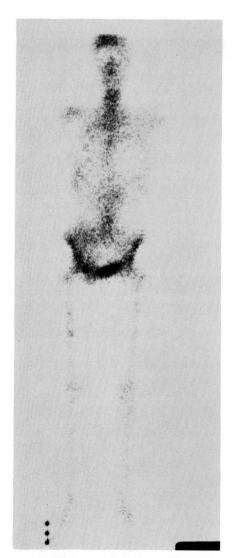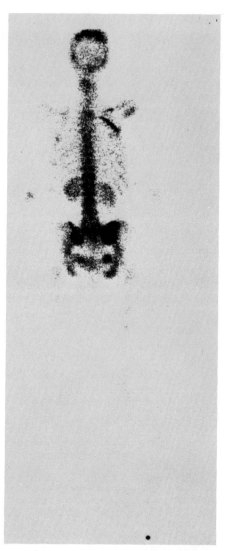

Fig. 5-6A. Anterior and posterior 99mTc diphosphonate bone scans
show areas of increased uptake in the skull, S-I joints, right pubic
bone and posterior right chest. This latter finding was interpreted
as being either in the scapula or a posterior rib. Radiographic
study revealed the lesion to be in the rib. The need for
correlation with radiographic studies is important since scanning is
not as anatomically specific, although more sensitive then
roentgenograms. The patient had a modified left mastectomy with
post operative radiation therapy. Note the decreased localization
of bone agent in the left anterior chest associated with radiation
therapy.

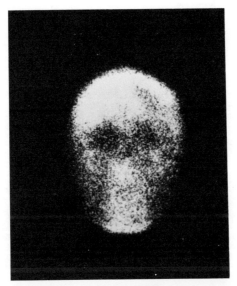

ANTERIOR

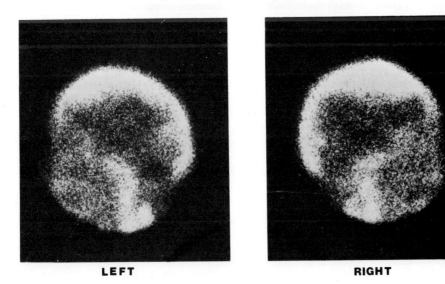

LEFT   **RIGHT**

Fig. 5-6B. Camera images (anterior, left, and right lateral) show
the skull lesions with a greater degree of resolution than the
rectilinear views. Compare anterior camera with anterior
rectilinear image.

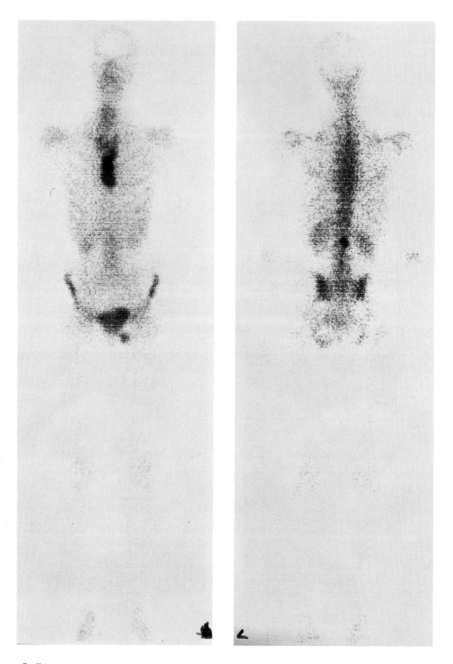

Fig. 5-7A. Initial anterior and posterior bone scan of this patient
shows sternal uptake as well as an abnormal area of uptake in the
lumbar spine. The focal activity noted beneath the bladder on the
anterior view represents urine contamination.

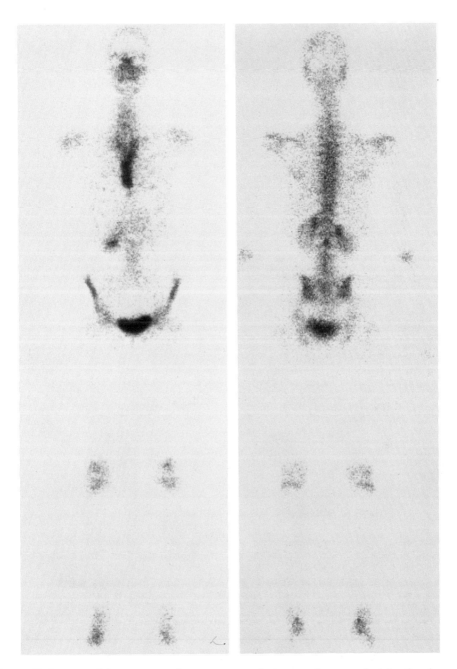

Fig. 5-7B. Follow-up study one year later, shows relatively less
intense activity in the sternum and lumbar spine.

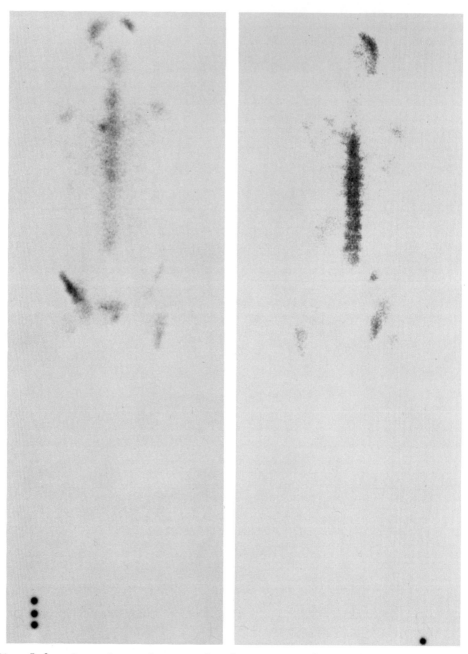

Fig. 5-8. Anterior and posterior bone scan of a patient with severe
skeletal metastatic disease. Note less than normal uptake in the
kidneys and no visualization of the soft tissues of the extremities.
This may be partly due to preferential uptake by the large amount of
skeletal tumor present.

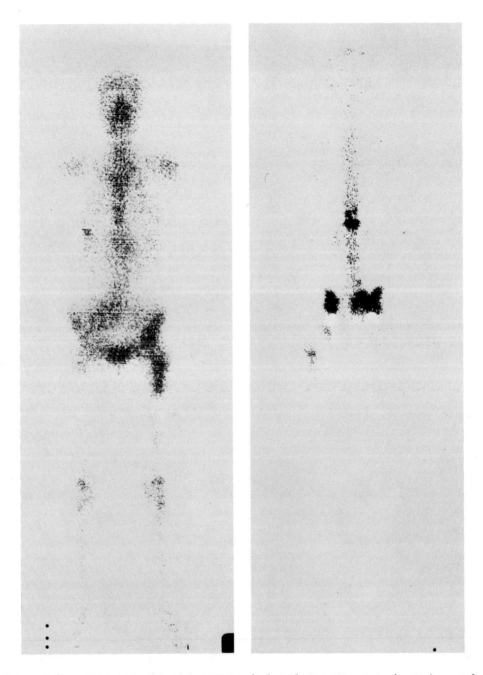

Fig. 5-9. Patient with extensive skeletal metastases. Anterior and posterior bone scan shows minimal soft tissue and renal localization.

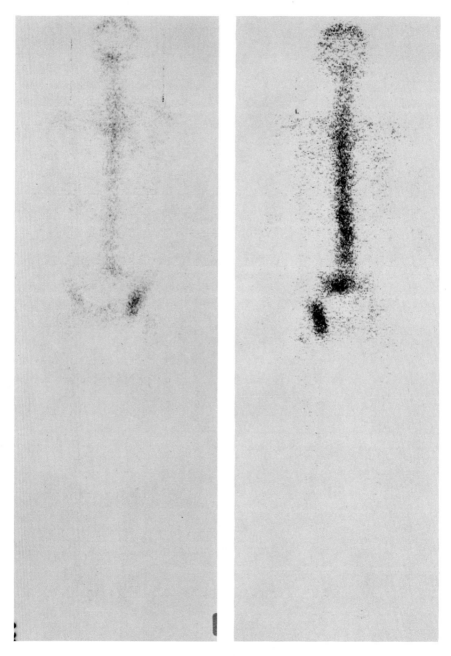

Fig. 5-10A. Anterior and posterior fluorine-18 skeletal scans reveal abnormal uptake in the sacrum and left ischium.

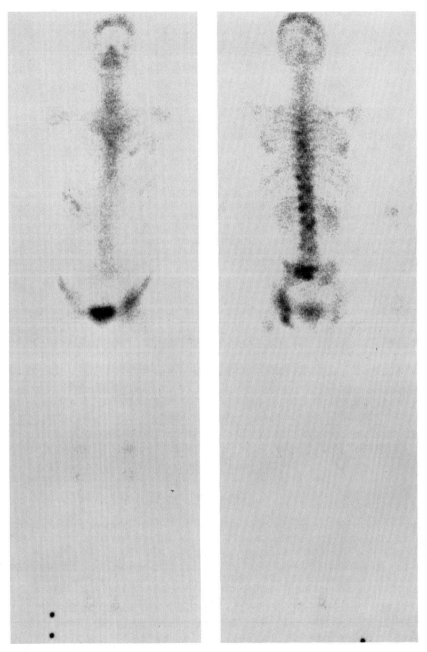

Fig. 5-10B. Study done with 99mTc polyphosphate within two months of the preceding fluorine-18 study shows far better detail and demonstrates several vertebral body lesions not visualized on the fluorine-18 scan.

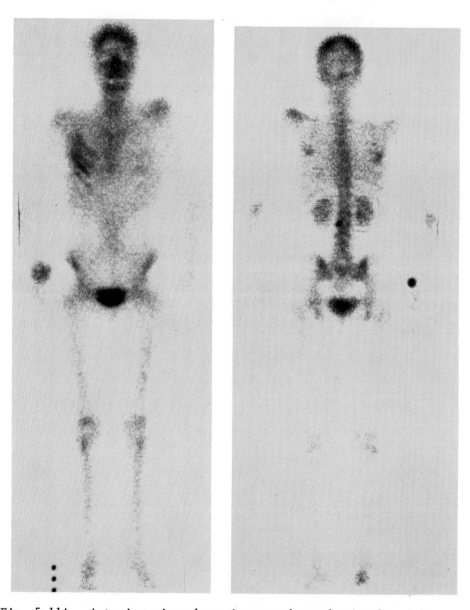

Fig. 5-11A. Anterior view shows increased uptake in the right upper
chest. This was the site of a recent mastectomy and therefore could
represent post-surgical changes or rib lesions. This area remained
unchanged on several serial scans leaving the differential diagnosis
unresolved. Rib radiographs were normal. Posterior view shows
increased uptake in the region of L-2 vertebral body. Increased
accumulation in the left shoulder was due to a chronic bursitis.

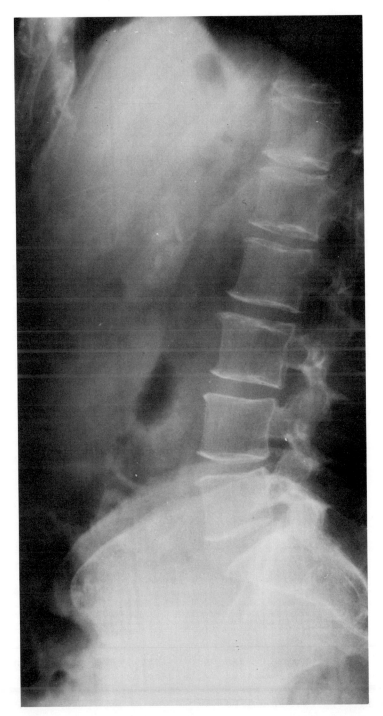

Fig. 5-11B. The radiograph of the spine was normal.

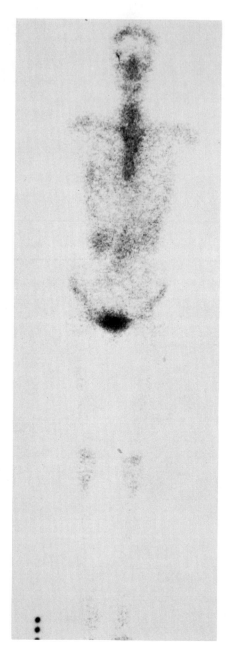

Fig. 5-12. This anterior scan shows slightly increased right chest
wall uptake which was believed to be secondary to the patient's
previous mastectomy. No areas of discrete increased uptake are seen,
thus making rib lesions unlikely.

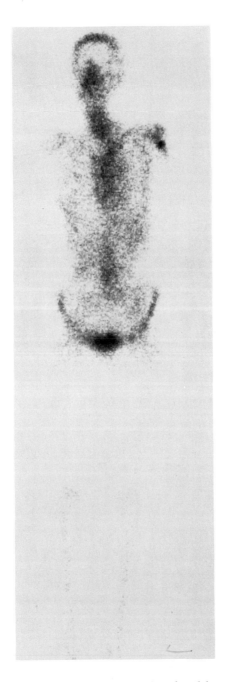

Fig. 5-13. Increased uptake in the left shoulder is secondary to recent trauma to the area. No metastases were identified on x-ray and the shoulder was normal on follow-up scan nine months later.

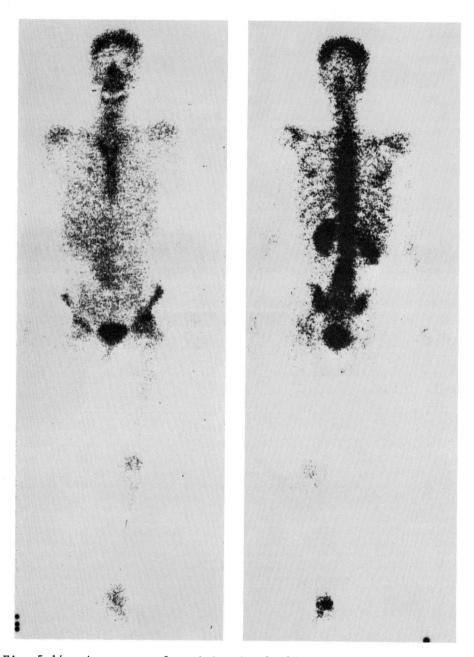

Fig. 5-14. Asymmetry of activity in the hip is present with less activity on the right side. This is due to poliomyelitis with right hemiatrophy. Left pelvic bone metastases, which might be suspected, were not present.

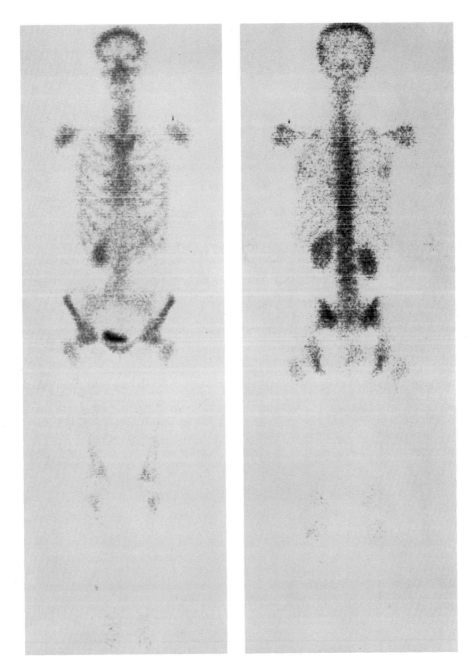

Fig. 5-15A. Anterior and posterior whole body bone scan showing uniform osseous localization of radionuclide with no skeletal asymmetry.

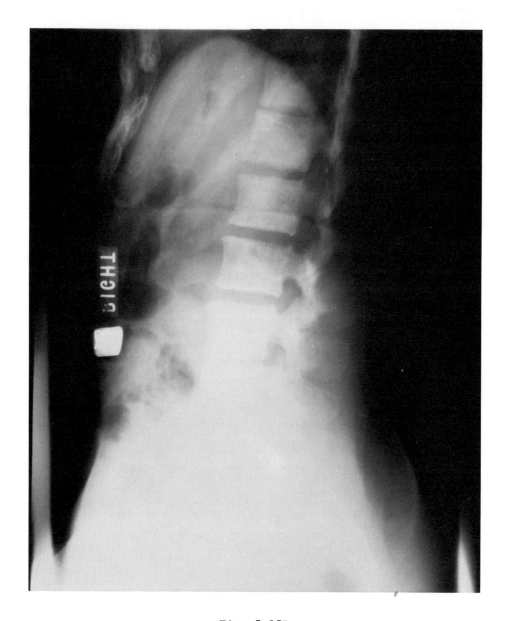

Fig. 5-15B

Fig. 5-15B,C,D. Metastases were found throughout the thoracic and
lumbar spine, ribs, pelvis, and femurs.

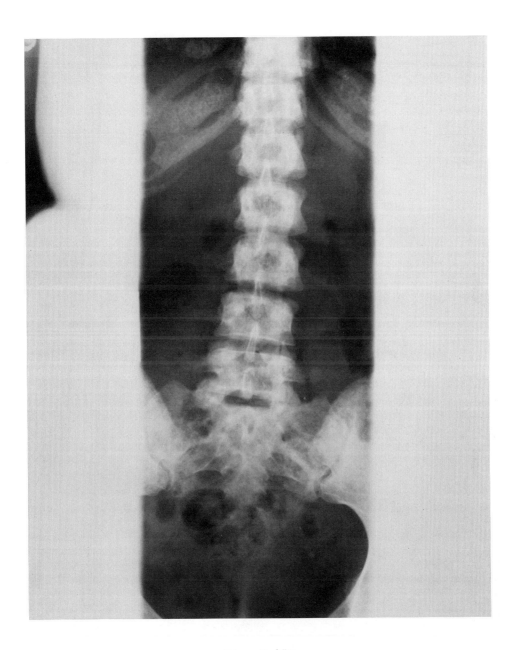

Fig. 5-15C

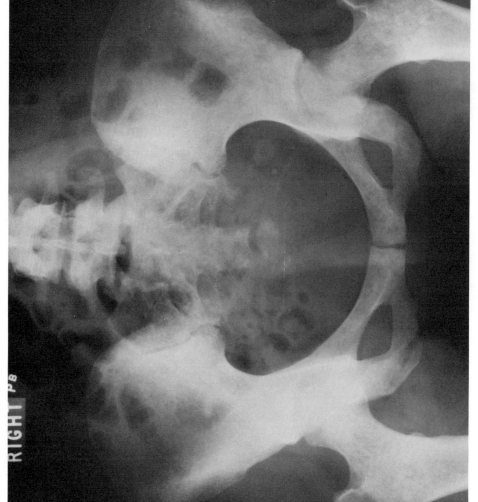

Fig. 5-15D

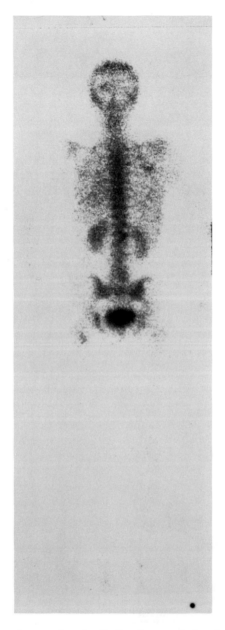

Fig. 5-16. Increased uptake in left femoral head is seen in this posterior bone scan. It corresponded in location to a bone island on the radiograph. The importance of correlating all scans with corresponding radiographs is obvious in order to avoid calling a benign bone lesion a metastasis.

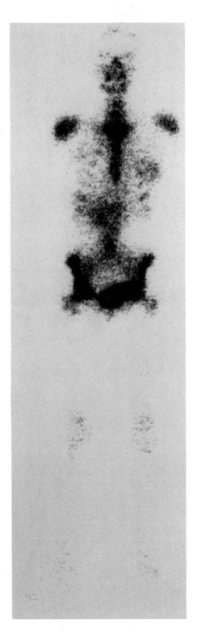

Fig. 5-17. This patient has a history of a right mastectomy one
year prior to her present admission. The anterior 99mTc
diphosphonate scan shows uptake of nuclide in the remaining left
breast. Clinically and at surgery, the patient has a second
carcinoma in this breast.

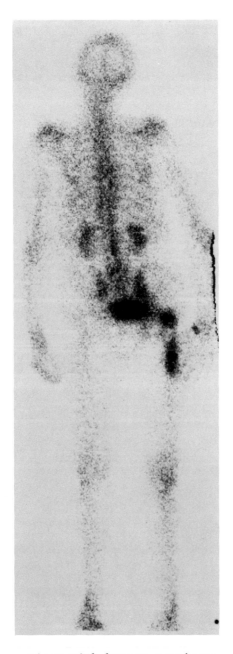

Fig. 5-18. A male patient with breast carcinoma. Posterior skeletal scintiscan shows increased uptake in the right femoral head and proximal femur. Originally interpreted as representing metastatic disease, this was proven to be Paget's disease by radiographic correlation.

References Chapter 5

1. Weber, D.A., Keyes, J.W., Jr., Benedetto, W.J., Wilson, G.A.
    Tc99m pyrophosphate for diagnostic bone imaging. Radiology 113:
    131, 1974.

2. Penelegrass, H.P., Potsaid M.S., Castronovo, F.P. The clinical
    use of 99mTc diphosphonate: a new agent for skeletal imagery.
    Radiology 107: 557, 1973.

3. Hosain, P. Technetium-99m labelled pyrophosphate: a simple and
    reproducible bone scanning agent. Radiology 111: 255, 1974.

4. Fletcher, J.W., Solaric-George E., Henry, R.E., Donati, R.M.
    Evaluation of 99mTc pyrophosphate as a bone imaging agent.
    Radiology 109: 467, 1973.

5. Silberstein, E.B., Saenger, E.L. Tofe, A.J.,
    Alexander, G.W., Jr., and Park, H.M. Imaging of bone metastases
    with 99mTc-Sn EHDP (diphosphonate), 18F, and skeletal radiography:
    a comparison of sensitivity. Radiology 107: 551, 1973.

6. Bachman, A.L., Sproul, E.E. Correlation of radiographic, autopsy
    findings in suspected metastases in the spine. Bull N Y Acad Med
    31: 146, 1955.

7. Edelstyn, G.A., Gillespie, P.J., Greball, F. The radiological
    demonstration of osseous metastases. Clin Radiol 18: 158, 1967.

8. Galasko, C.S.B. The detection of skeletal metastases from
    mammary cancer by gamma camera scintigraphy. Brit J Surg 56:
    757, 1969.

9. Galasko, C.S.B. Skeletal metastases and mammary cancer. Ann R
    Coll Surg Eng 50: 3, 1972.

10. Rubin, P., Ciccio, S. Status of bone scanning for bone metastases
    in breast cancer. Cancer 24: 1338, 1969.

11. Sklaroff, D.M., Charkes, N.D. Bone metastases from breast cancer
    at the time of radical mastectomy. Surg Gynec Obstet 127: 763,
    1968.

12. Hoffman, H.C., Marty, R. Bone scanning: Its value in the
    preoperative evaluation of patients with suspicious breast
    Masses. Am J Surg 124: 194, 1972.

13. Hopkins, G.B., Kristensen, K.A.B. Whole body skeletal
    scintiphotography in the detection of occult breast carcinomas.
    Calif Med 119: 10, 1973.

14. Charkes, N.D., Young, I., Sklaroff, D.M. The pathologic basis
    of the strontium bone scan. JAMA 206: 2482, 1968.

15. Frankel, R.S., Richman, S.D., Levenson, S.M., Nelson, R.L.,
    Ingle, J.N., Tormey, D.C., Jones, A.E., Johnston, G.S. Bone
    scintigraphy in breast carcinoma. J Nucl Med 15: 491, 1974.

16. Frankel, R.S., Jones, A.E., Cohen, J.A., Johnson, K.W.,
    Johnston, G.S., Pomeroy, T.C. Clinical conditions of 67Ga and
    skeletal whole body radionuclide studies with radiography in
    Ewing's sarcoma. Radiology 110: 597, 1974.

17. Jones, A.E., Frankel, R.S., Di Chiro, G., Johnston, G.S. Brain
    scintigraphy with 99mTc pertechnetate, 99mTc polyphosphate, and
    67Ga citrate. Radiology 112: 123, 1974.

18. Frankel, R.S., Johnson, K.W., Mabry, J.J., Johnston, G.S.
    "Normal" bone radionuclide image with diffuse skeletal lymphoma.
    A case report. Radiology 111: 365, 1974.

19. Thripkaew, A.K., Henkin, R.E., Quinn, J.L., III, False negative
    bone scans in disseminated metastatic disease. Radiology 113:
    383, 1974.

20. Hattner, R.S., Miller, S.W., Schimmel, D. Significance of renal
    asymmetry in bone scans: Experience in 795 cases. J Nucl Med
    16: 161, 1975.

21. Sharma, S.M., Quinn, J.L, III, Significance of 18 F-fluoride
    renal accumulation during bone imaging. J Nucl Med 13: 744,
    1972.

Gallium-67 Scintigraphy

Steven D. Richman, M.D.

Department of Nuclear Medicine
National Institutes of Health
Bethesda, Maryland

It has long been the ambition of nuclear medicine to provide a direct, tumor specific scanning agent, that has a specific affinity for neoplastic tissue. Thus far gallium-67 citrate (67Ga) is the tumor-seeking radionuclide which has achieved the greatest clinical success. Intensive investigations have demonstrated that a wide spectrum of neoplasms concentrate 67Ga to varying degrees (1,2)(Fig. 6-15).

Gallium-67, however, has proved a relatively insensitive agent for the detection of primary breast carcinoma. Higasi (3) studied 16 cases of breast carcinoma and eight were positive with 67Ga scintigraphy. Among nine patients with breast carcinoma, Langhammer (4) demonstrated only three with abnormal concentration of 67Ga. Lavender (5) was able to show increased 67Ga activity in two of ten primary malignancies. Five of seven patients had increased uptake in the series reported by Fogh (6). Our studies show a disappointing 52% detection rate for primary adenocarcinoma of the breast in 21 patients evaluated with 67Ga. Gallium-67 is not particularly suited to gamma camera scintigraphy and special breast views have not improved its diagnostic usefulness (see Chapter 4). Furthermore, several pitfalls in interpretation are encountered (Figs. 6-3,4). The complicating factor of physiologic 67Ga concentration in the prelactating and lactating breast is well documented (6,7). Women on cyclic hormones have demonstrated increased mammary uptake (8). Normal diffuse uptake might therefore mask a focal, pathologic accumulation. "False-positive" localization can occur, albeit infrequently, in fibrocystic breast disease (Figs. 6-3C,4B) and gynecomastia (3,9,10).

Gallium-67 is no substitute for roentgenographic examination of breast disease, and the search for an effective breast scanning agent continues. The role of 67Ga, however, need not be relegated to the preoperative evaluation of the primary tumor. We have studied 67Ga scintigraphy as a diagnostic adjunct in 104 patients either after mastectomy, or in inoperable cases, before therapy.

Whole body 67Ga scintigraphy was routinely performed 48-72 hours after intravenous administration of 35-50 uCi/kg body weight of 67Ga. A dual probe 5 inch crystal whole body scanner with 5:1 minification and a spectrometer window setting of 130-330KeV was used. Adequate bowel preparation to eliminate interfering 67Ga from the abdomen was necessary for accurate interpretation.

Eighty-three patients with evidence for metastatic breast carcinoma were studied. Gallium-67 proved less sensitive than skeletal scintigraphy for the detection of osseous metastases (Figs. 6-6,7,8,20). Corroboration of skeletal involvement occurred in 34 (65%) of 52 cases. In patients with multiple bony metastases, 67Ga often failed to concentrate in all sites of tumor. When both 67Ga and 99mTc diphosphonate were positive the bone lesions were better visualized with the latter agent (Fig. 6-8). In only two cases with known multiple metastases, did 67Ga identify an additional skeletal metastasis before either bone scintigraphy or roentgenogram examinations.

Gallium-67 failed to localize differentially in 20 of 25 cases with secondary hepatic neoplasm (Figs. 6-9,11,12). Twenty of these patients had focal defects on the 99mTc sulfur colloid liver scan. In two cases, metastatic tumor resulted in areas of preferential 67Ga localization corresponding with areas of diminished colloid uptake. Two patients had decreased 67Ga activity in the region of large liver scan defects. One patient with severe hepatic replacement had absent 67Ga uptake throughout the liver parenchyma (Fig. 6-11).

The accuracy of 67Ga for lung metastases was also disappointing; seven (35%) of 20 cases with roentgenographic evidence of pulmonary involvement had abnormal 67Ga uptake (Figs. 6-13,14).

With regard to individual organ tracer techniques, the 67Ga scan played a limited confirmatory role in the assessment of metastatic lesions. For serial follow-up of metastatic tumor, bone, brain, and liver scans consistently provided information far superior to the 67Ga scan. Occasionally 67Ga uptake provided an ancillary visual index of tumor involvement and was used in conjunction with isolated organ studies and roentgenographic examination.

In some patients with known metastatic tumor, 67Ga scintigraphy did demonstrate a unique diagnostic value. The detection of mediastinal involvement in eight cases (10%) of this select population was most rewarding (Figs. 6-5,6,16). Autopsy in two patients confirmed metastatic breast carcinoma. Mediastinoscopy, utilized to obtain tissue for hormone-receptor studies, was positive for metastatic breast carcinoma in four of five patients undergoing this procedure. In three biopsy-proven cases, 67Ga was the sole means of detection of mediastinal tumor in the presence of unremarkable chest roentgenograms and tomograms of the mediastinum.

Gallium-67 scintigraphy was performed in 21 post-surgical patients in whom all other parameters indicated a disease-free status. Gallium-67 scanning provided a useful, objective procedure corroborating the absence of metastases in 20 cases. Although 67Ga scans were negative in 20 of the patients, in one instance 67Ga demonstrated occult mediastinal tumor as the only evidence for metastasis. Therapy was instituted and the follow-up 67Ga scan returned to normal.

Gallium-67 scanning is a limited corroborative modality in both primary and metastatic breast carcinoma. Gallium-67 scanning cannot replace organ-specific radionuclide studies nor available clinical, laboratory and roentgenographic indices of tumor involvement. However, 67Ga has been most valuable for the detection of mediastinal breast metastases. Since documentation of the total extent and activity of metastatic disease is important for prognosis and therapy, the 67Ga scan scan can contribute useful information especially in breast carcinoma patients with known metastatic disease. Judicious use of 67Ga scintigraphy is recommended in the preoperative patient and as a screening procedure in postoperative patients without other evidence for metastases.

Finally, the propensity of 67Ga to concentrate in inflammatory lesions can be of considerable clinical value (11,12) since 67Ga has been used successfully to localize and follow inflammatory processes in the septic patient (Fig. 6-20) with breast carcinoma.

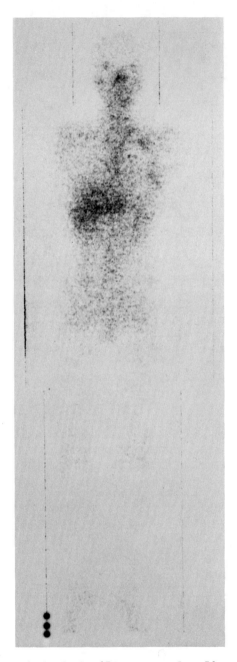

Fig. 6-1. Anterior whole body 67Ga scan of a 51 year-old woman
with carcinoma of the left breast. The scan shows increased 67Ga
uptake in the primary tumor. There is also increased activity in
the left axillary region. Radical mastectomy was performed and 25
of 26 nodes were positive for metastases.

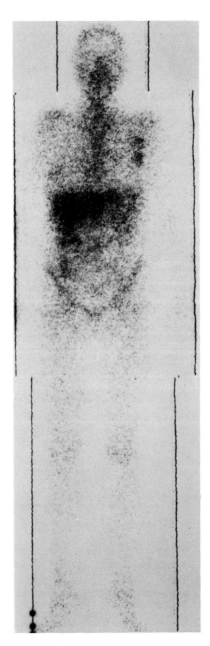

Fig. 6-2. A 62 year-old woman with inoperable adenocarcinoma of the left breast and extension into the left axilla. Increased 67Ga activity is shown in the primary tumor, the left axilla and the right breast. Mammography demonstrated only fibrocystic disease in the right breast, but clinical examination confirmed metastatic involvement.

Fig. 6-3A. Pitfalls in interpretation, diffuse breast activity:
Intense 67Ga activity, in a post-partum lactating patient with
lymphoma. Note abnormal inguinal nodes.

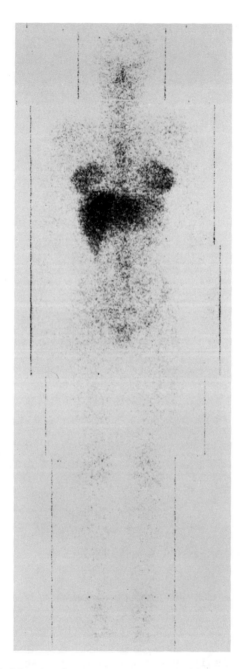

Fig. 6-3B. Pitfalls in interpretation, diffuse breast activity:
Physiologic breast activity in a 21 year-old woman taking birth
control pills. There was no evidence for breast disease.

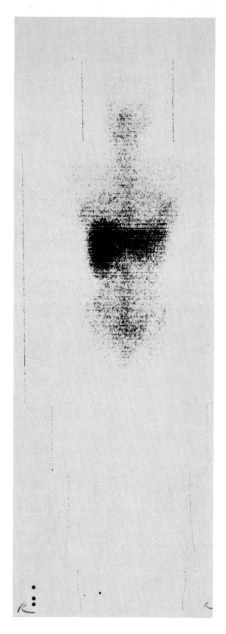

Fig. 6-3C. Pitfalls in interpretation, diffuse breast activity:
Diffuse mammary uptake in a 39 year-old patient with fibrocystic
disease of the right breast and a fibroadenoma in the left breast.

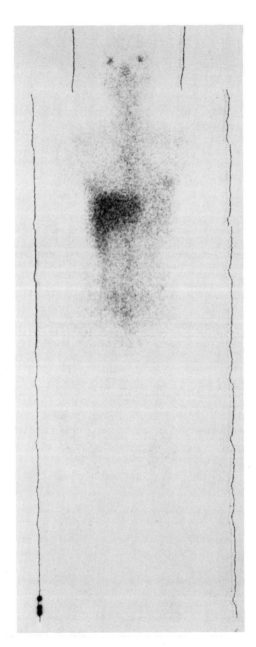

Fig. 6-3D. Adenocarcinoma of the right breast in a 41 year-old
woman. Mammography indicated a malignancy. Bilateral, diffuse
breast uptake would obscure any focal 67Ga abnormality.

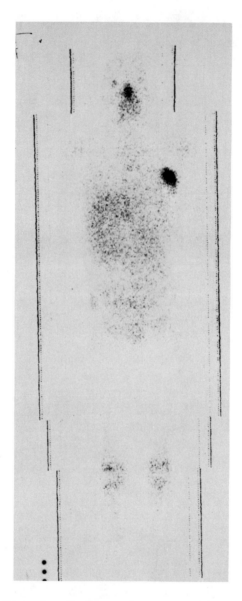

Fig. 6-4A. Pitfalls, focal abnormality: Discrete activity in left
breast of a 15 year-old girl with acute myeloblastic leukemia.
Biopsy revealed a myeloblastoma. (Intense nasopharyngeal 67Ga
activity represents an abnormal mass as well).

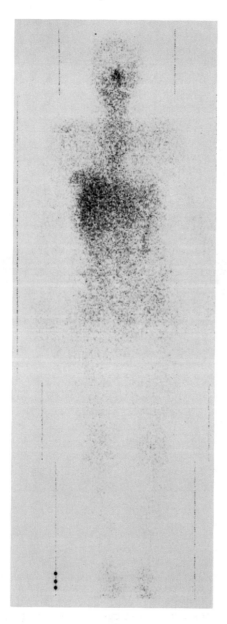

Fig. 6-4B. Pitfalls, focal abnormality: Focal activity
representing fibrocystic disease in the right breast of a 50
year-old woman. Left radical mastectomy was performed one year
prior to the 67Ga scan. Clinical examination of the right breast
was normal and mammography showed only minimal fibrocystic change.

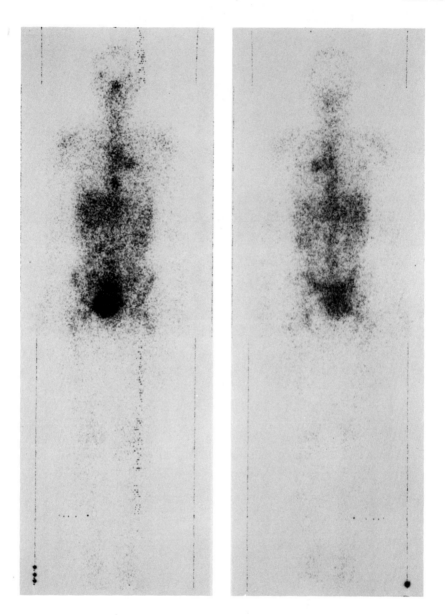

Fig. 6-5. The patient is a 31 year-old woman with bilateral
mastectomies. Bone scan and roentgenographic examination of the
sternum demonstrated lytic metastases. Anterior and posterior 67Ga
views showed sternal metastases and also demonstrated abnormal
uptake in the left hilum. Chest roentgenograms and tomography were
unremarkable. Mediastinoscopy was positive for metastatic breast
carcinoma. (Artifact is seen in the left leg and external to the
skull).

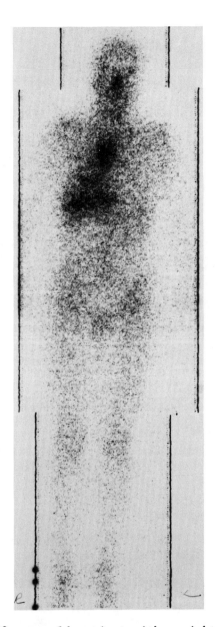

Fig. 6-6A. This 62 year-old patient with a right radical mastectomy and evidence for bone and skin metastases also has metastatic disease in the mediastinum. Gallium-67 failed to localize in the known metastases, but revealed mediastinal tumor in this previously unsuspected site of involvement.

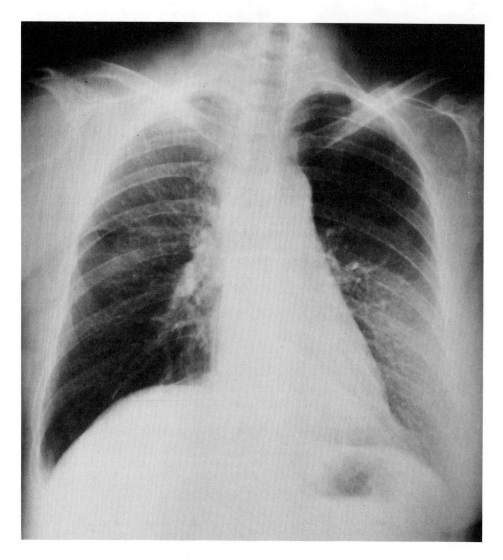

Fig. 6-6B. Chest roentgenogram and tomography failed to disclose
the mediastinal tumors.

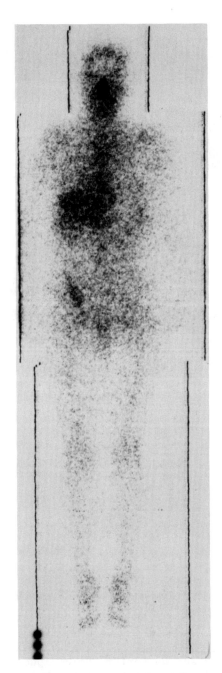

Fig. 6-6C. Following combination chemotherapy the 67Ga scan reverted to normal.

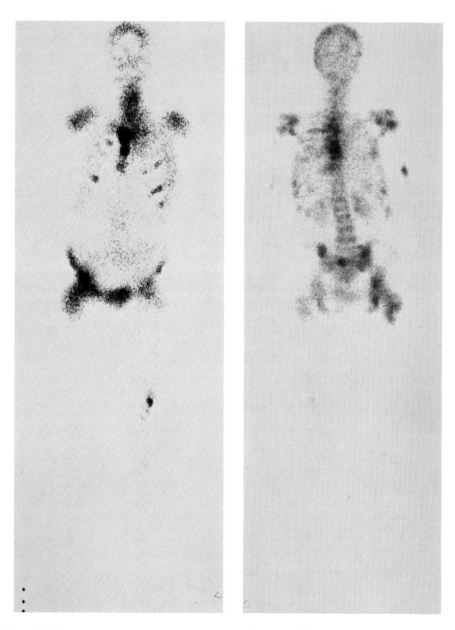

Fig. 6-7A. Anterior and posterior 99mTc diphosphonate bone scan
demonstrates multiple sites of metastatic breast carcinoma.

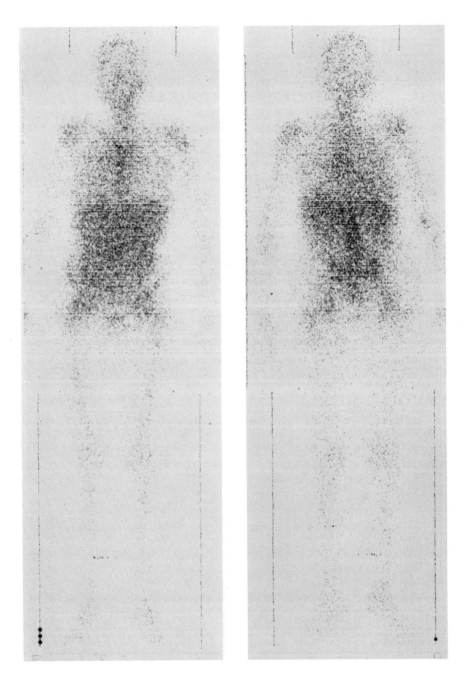

Fig. 6-7B. Anterior and posterior 67Ga scan failed to identify any bony metastases.

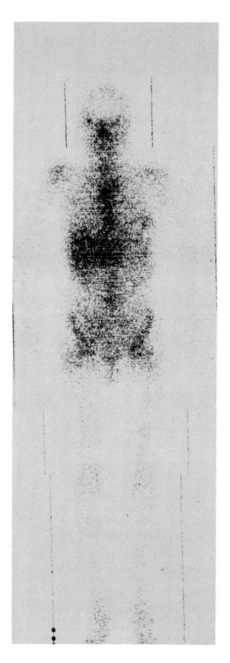

Fig. 6-8A. Anterior 67Ga shows questionable faint abnormal tracer in the sternum and left lower rib cage.

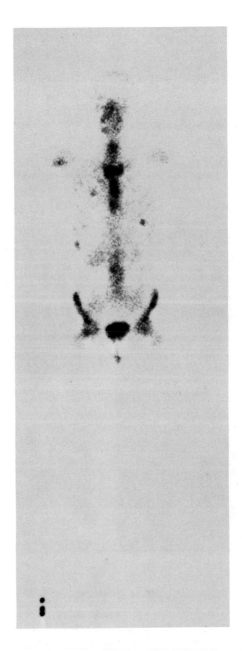

Fig. 6-8B. The bone scan with 99mTc diphosphonate reveals more intense uptake in the corresponding regions and demonstrates additional metastases in the right shoulder, right rib cage and in the right hip.

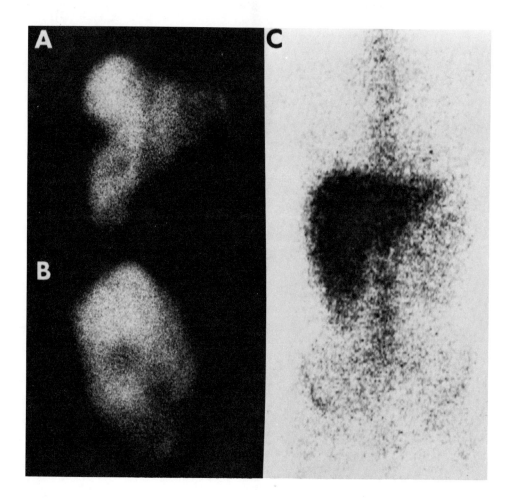

Fig. 6-9. Biopsy proven metastatic breast carcinoma involving the
liver of a 31 year-old woman. Scintigraphy reveals hepatomegaly
and large focal defects A) anterior, B) right lateral. Gallium-67
scan shows enlargement but no hepatic metastases are apparent (C).

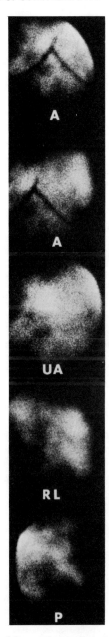
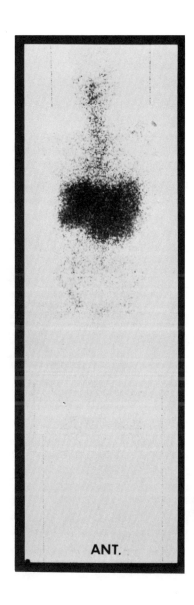

Fig. 6-10. There is increased 67Ga activity seen on the anterior
whole body view in the right lobe of the liver which corresponds
with the region of decreased liver activity on the 99mTc sulfur
colloid views. Secondary hepatic neoplasm accounted for
parenchymal replacement (Gamma camera images from top:
A = reclining view with rib markers; A = reclining view
including left hepatic lobe with rib markers; UA = upright
anterior; RL = upright right lateral; P = upright posterior).

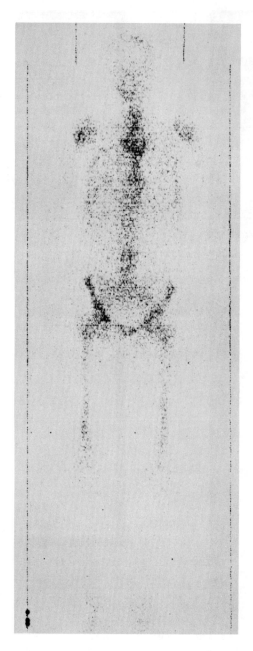

Fig. 6-11. Anterior whole body 67Ga scan of a 37 year-old patient with a previous right mastectomy and severe liver replacement by metastases. There is no 67Ga uptake by the liver. Well defined bony concentration, in part, reflects widely disseminated osseous metastases.

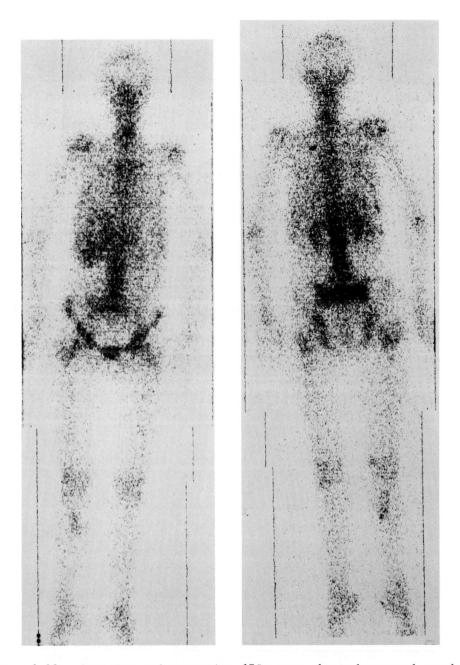

Fig. 6-12. Anterior and posterior 67Ga scan shows decreased uptake in the right lobe of the liver in a patient with marked hepatic failure. Multiple bony metastases are present. Note the renal route of excretion. Kidneys were free of tumor at autopsy.

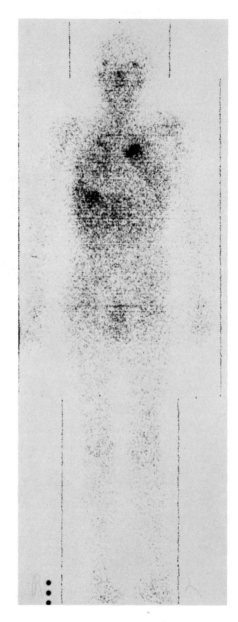

Fig. 6-13. Gallium-67 uptake in the right lower and left upper lung fields in a 65 year-old woman with a right radical mastectomy and pulmonary metastases. Gallium-67 abnormalities corresponded with large lung nodules. Liver biopsy was normal.

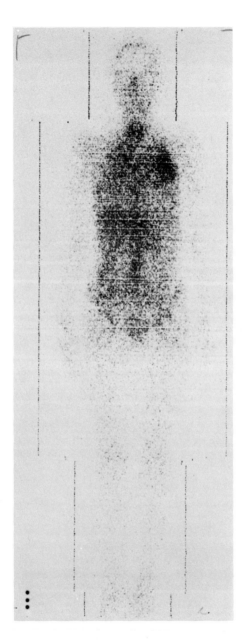

Fig. 6-14. Increased 67Ga uptake throughout both lungs accurately
confirmed diffuse pulmonary metastases.

Fig. 6-15. Two years prior to admission this 38
year-old woman had an excisional biopsy for
infiltrating ductal carcinoma in the right breast.
At that time, abdominal exploration for a pelvic
mass revealed a cystic papillary serous
cystadenocarcinoma of the right ovary. A right
paratracheal mass discovered on chest
roentgenogram prompted a clinical work-up.
Gallium-67 scan confirmed the chest tumor.
Thoracotomy revealed metastatic ovarian carcinoma
and appropriate treatment was instituted. This
case demonstrates the non-specificity of 67Ga
uptake.

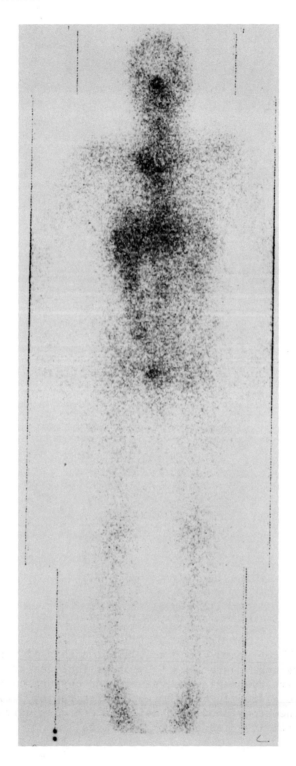

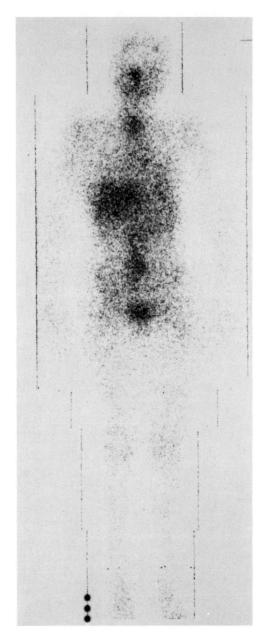

Fig. 6-16. Three years prior to admission this 55 year-old woman
had a left radical mastectomy. Symptoms included at the time of
this study were dysphagia, hoarseness and dyspnea on exertion.
Gallium-67 localized in the thoracic inlet region. Biopsy at the
time of tracheostomy confirmed metastatic breast carcinoma.
(Abdominal activity cleared with laxatives.)

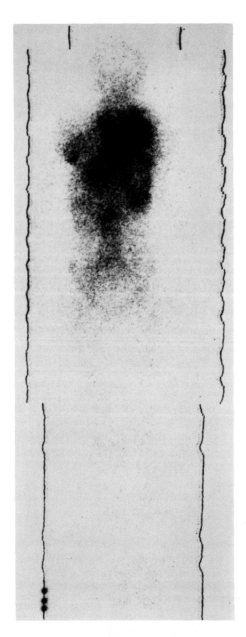

Fig. 6-17. Anterior scan of a 56 year-old woman with intense
uptake in a massive, fixed, left breast tumor involving both chest
walls and bilateral axillary regions.

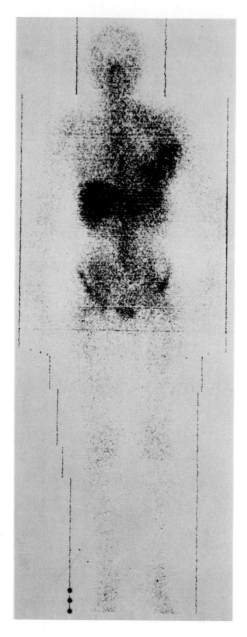

Fig. 6-18. Seven years after a right radical mastectomy this 53 year-old woman presented with disseminated metastases. There is 67Ga localization in the left breast, left axilla, and left supraclavicular nodes. Abnormal iliac activity represents bony metastases.

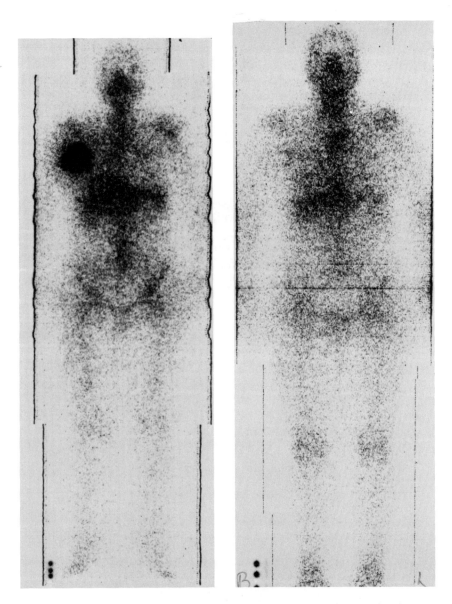

Fig. 6-19. A large inflammatory carcinoma of the right breast with intense 67Ga is seen in this study (left). After effective therapy the lesion improved clinically and 67Ga scan returned to normal (right).

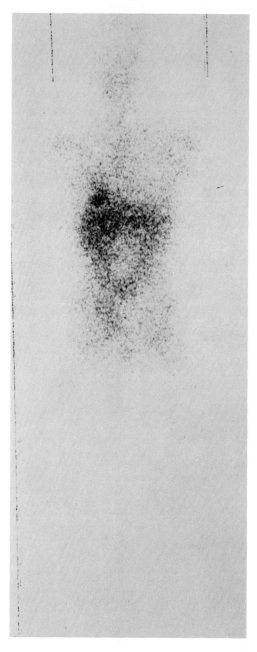

Fig. 6-20. Three weeks after surgery 67Ga localized in an infected mastectomy site, but failed to demonstrate known bony metastases.

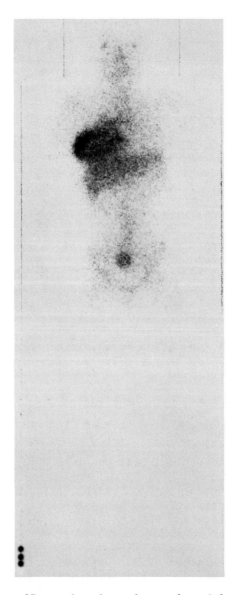

Fig. 6-21. Gallium-67 uptake throughout the right breast of this
35 year-old woman two months after left mastectomy. The patient
was lactating in the post-operative period (prolactin levels were
elevated). Persistent focal activity in the pelvis represents 67Ga
uptake in an asymptomatic uterine fibroid confirmed at the time of
oophorectomy.

References Chapter 6

1. Edwards, C.L., Hayes, R.L. Localization of tumors with
    radiosotopes. (In) Clinical Uses of Radionuclides: Critical
    Comparison with Other Techniques. Oak Ridge, Tennessee, 618,
    1971.

2. Johnston, G.S., Jones, A.E. Atlas of Gallium 67 Scintigraphy.
    New York, Plenum Press, 1973.

3. Higasi, T., Nakayama, Y., Murata, A., Nakamure, K., Sugiyama, M.,
    Kawaguchi, T., Suzuki, S. Clinical evaluation of 67Ga
    citrate scanning. J Nucl Med 13: 196, 1972.

4. Langhammer, H., Glaubitt, G., Grebe, S.F., Hampe, J.F.,
    Haubold, U., Hor, G., Kaul, S., Keoppe, P., Koppenhagen, J.,
    Roedler, H.D., van der Schoot, J.B. 67Ga for tumor scanning
    J Nucl Med 13: 25, 1972.

5. Lavender, J.P., Lowe, J., Barker, J.R., Burn, J.I., Chauhdri, M.A.
    Gallium 67 citrate scanning in neoplastic and inflammatory .
    lesions. Brit J Radiol 44: 361, 1971.

6. Fogh, J. 67Ga accumulation in malignant tumors and in the pre-
    lacting or lactating breast. Pro Soc Exp Biol Med 138: 1086,
    1971.

7. Larson, S.M., Schall, G.L. Gallium 67 concentration in
    human breast milk. JAMA 218: 257, 1971.

8. Larson, S.M., Milder, M.S., Johnston, G.S. Interpretation
    of the 67Ga photoscan. J Nucl Med 14: 208, 1973.

9. Richman, S.D., Brodey, P.A., Frankel, R.S., de Moss, E.V.,
    Tormey, D.C., Johnston, G.S. Breast scintigraphy with
    99mTc pertechnetate and 67Ga citrate. J Nucl Med
    16: 293, 1975.

10. Winchell, H.S., Sanchez, P.D., Watanabe, C.K., Hollander, L.,
    Anger, H.O., McRae, J. Visualization of tumors in humans
    using 67Ga citrate and the Anger whole body scanner,
    scintillation camera and tomographic scanner. J Nucl Med 11:
    459, 1970.

11. Harvey, W.C., Poduluff, D.A., Kopp, D.T. 67Gallium in 68
    consecutive infection searches. J. Nucl. Med 16: 2, 1975.

12. Littenberg, R.L., Taketa, R.M., Alazraki, N., et al. Gallium
    67 for localization of septic lesions. Ann Intern Med 79:
    403, 1973.

CHAPTER 7

Radiologic Evaluation:
Roentgenographic and Other Procedures

George S. Flinn, M.D., Robert S. Francis, M.D.,
Stanley M. Levenson, M.D.

Department of Radiology, Clinical Center
Department of Nuclear Medicine, Clinical Center
National Institutes of Health
Bethesda, Maryland

The contribution of diagnostic radiology in the initial
detection and follow-up of patients with carcinoma of the breast (1)
is well accepted. Techniques and procedures used in the
radiographic evaluation of patients with suspected or established
carcinoma of the breast have become routine diagnostic methods in
this disease. Thermography and ultrasonography are being evaluated
as aids in breast cancer diagnosis in many radiology departments. A
common sequence of application of these methods includes:

Breast Evaluation

Mammography and Xeroradiography: Conventional film mammography
(2,3,4) and xeroradiography (5) are the most reliable studies in the
evaluation of suspicious breast masses (Figs. 7-1, 7-2, 7-3).
However, the role of mammography in large-scale screening of
asymptomatic patients has yet to be defined. Only after long-term
prospective surveys have provided adequate data can valid
recommendations be made on the optimum type and frequency of x-ray
examination and patient selection.

Until recently, a usual policy has been to perform both
conventional low killivolt (KV), high MAS (milliampsec) non-screen
film mammograms along with xeroradiographs during the initial
evaluation of a patient with a breast tumor. In follow-up studies,
only mammograms were utilized. Presently, however, in an effort to
reduce the patient radiation dose (6) and simplify the procedure,
xeroradiography is used exclusively. This is accomplished with a
1.0 mm focal spot tungsten tube interfaced to a single phase, full

wave rectified generator and inherent aluminum filtration.
Tube-film distance is 30-36 inches. Exposure factors in the
positive mode are 33-42 KV at 400-450 MAS. Craniocaudad and
mediolateral views are routinely obtained. The axilla is usually
well visualized on the mediolateral view, obviating additional
axillary images. Compression on the craniocaudad view is obtained
by inserting an inflated balloon into the "mouth" of a long cone.
The balloon is firm and exerts adequate pressure on the breast
without causing discomfort. Conventional mammography is rarely
used, as only occasional cases have been seen where
microcalcifications were more easily visualized on mammograms than
on xeroradiographs.

The indications for mammography are quite broad with the aim
being to differentiate a benign breast process from malignant
disease. The following are indications for mammography:

1. Patients presenting with breast masses, pain or nipple
    discharge.
2. The baseline examination of the "lumpy" breast.
3. Large breasts in patients with a new breast complaint (large
    breasts can prevent palpation of a cancer easily seen
    on mammograms).
4. A screening or localizing procedure prior to breast
    biopsy.
5. Confirmation of clinical breast cancer.
6. Evaluation of the remaining breast for carcinoma after
    mastectomy, (This high risk group of patients comprises
    a large percentage of patients with mammograms at our
    institution.
7. Family history of breast carcinoma. These patients have a
    2-3 fold increased incidence of breast carcinoma.
8. Unknown primary cancer and metastases in an adult female.

Thermography: Thermography is another technique for breast
examination (7,8,9,10). The thermogram registers the heat pattern
of the breast via a monitor sensitive to infra-red radiation. The
increased metabolic rate of tumors causes increased heat production
resulting in an abnormal thermal pattern. Thermograms are easily
performed but difficult to interpret, and have a significant false-
positive rate of 15-20%. The inexact nature of the technique
precludes its use as a single mass screening procedure. The
thermogram is always used in conjunction with physical exam. When
there is an abnormal thermogram, supplemental mammography should be
obtained prior to breast biopsy.

Ultrasonography: Ultrasonographic examination of the breast

(11,12,13,14,15) is being evaluated as a screening procedure by many investigators, but is neither generally available, nor widely accepted. Its use in the examination of a breast mass is considered quite accurate in differentiating between cystic (Figs. 7-4) and solid breast lesions. The most accurate mode of ultrasound scanning for small lesions is the A-scan, although the B-scan is now being utilized with both cystic and solid lesions which are easily identified if the lesion is palpable. With improvements in instrumentation and further physician experience, ultrasonography appears to be a promising modality in screening for breast disease.

Detection of Metastases

Metastatic Survey: Because of the frequency of skeletal involvement, plain film radiographs of the axial and appendicular skeleton are used in conjunction with bone scans for the initial detection of bony metastases (16,17,18,19,20,21). The bone scan has been invaluable in isolating specific areas for special tomographic evaluation. Chapter 5 presents and describes the value of bone scintigraphy in patients with breast carcinoma.

The skeletal survey, the frequency of which is being re-evaluated in this patient population, is performed in the following manner. The routine metastatic survey includes AP and lateral projections of the lumbar and thoracic spine, lateral cervical spine, 3-view skull, AP pelvis including proximal femurs (Fig. 7-5A,B,C), PA and lateral chest, AP views of upper and lower extremities, and any indicated projections of symptomatic regions (Fig. 7-6). Rib detail views have been especially helpful in conjunction with suspicious bone scans. The bone survey has been useful in differentiating areas of degenerative or benign bone disease in the presence of an abnormal bone scan. Its particular value appears to be in the follow-up of skeletal metastases detected by skeletal scintigraphy (Fig. 7-7A,B,C,D,E,) and in determining response to chemotherapy.

Tomography: Tomographic examination of suspicious areas seen on plain films, e.g., the spine, in which the extent of involvement needs further definition, has become standard procedure. It is also quite common to perform tomography on the cervicothoracic junction, sacrum, sternum and other sites, which though not necessarily suspicious, are otherwise difficult to adequately define.

Full-lung tomography warrants significant consideration. A review of all full-lung tomograms performed over a one year period in our department demonstrated several cases of positive tomograms

with metastatic nodules. Corresponding radiographs were normal.
Full-lung tomography utilizing linear sweep in 1 cm. sections has
been of value in the initial evaluation and follow-up of metastatic
lung disease in breast carcinoma patients (Fig. 7-8A,B).

    Ultrasonography: Ultrasound examination of the liver
(22,23,24,25,26,27) using conventional bistable equipment is much
less sensitive than liver scintigraphy in the evaluation of hepatic
metastases (Fig. 7-9). Ultrasound can differentiate between cystic
and solid lesions in the liver, and this may well evolve to be the
prime value of the hepatic ultrasound examination. Another
potential use of this modality is the determination of temporal size
changes in metastatic liver lesions; some suggest that ultrasound
will supplant the routine liver scan for this purpose in the future.
In addition, focal "cold" areas noted on 99mTc sulfur colloid liver
scan may be evaluated by ultrasound examination. Intrahepatic
gallbladder and enlarged portal vein might be differentiated from
metastases by ultrasonography. At present,hepatic ultrasonography
isdifficult because of the interference of ribs when imaging the
liver.

    Special Procedures: The need for angiography occasionally
arises in the evaluation of metastatic disease. Carotid angiography
in patients with neurologic manifestations suggesting intracerebral
metastases can be helpful when the brain scan is positive or
equivocal. The availability of computerized axial tomography
(C.A.T.) for the evaluation of brain lesions may further modify
the approach to those patients now requiring carotid
angiography.

    Abdominal angiography is rarely necessary for evaluation of
visceral metastases. In the occasional patient with
gastrointestinal hemorrhage secondary to metastases or chemotherapy,
visceral angiography is helpful in localizing the site of bleeding.
Hemorrhaging can hopefully then be controlled by the selective
infusion of vasopressors or selective embolization of the bleeding
site.

    Myelography is often used to diagnose and localize the site of
spinal metastases. These are usually extradural deposits having
spread contiguously from bony metastases. The contrast material is
usually left in the subarachnoid space after the procedure to allow
radiographic visualization of tumor response to therapy.

    In summary, an overview of the radiographic, thermographic, and
ultrasonographic methods of evaluating patients with suspected or
proven breast carcinoma has been presented. No attempt has been made
to list all the possible radiographic modalities or to dogmatically

recommend their specific use. The ramifications of whole-body
C.A.T. scanning systems will certainly change the future application
of diagnostic radiology with hopeful benefit for patients with
breast carcinoma.

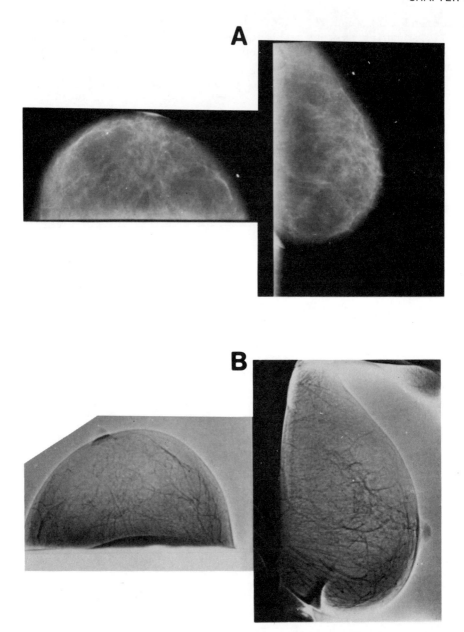

Fig. 7-1. Following radical mastectomy this 64 year old woman had mammographic (A) and xeroradiographic (B) examinations of her right breast. Minimal atrophic changes are seen in an otherwise unremarkable breast. (Note: For Figs. 7-1, 7-2, and 7-3, craniocaudad view appears on left and lateral view adjacent on right).

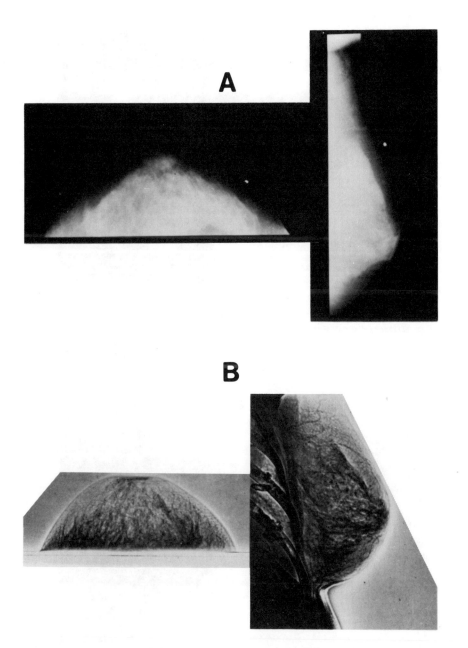

Fig. 7-2. Mammogram (A) and xeroradiogram (B) demonstrate fibrous
dysplasia in the remaining right breast of this 65 year old woman.

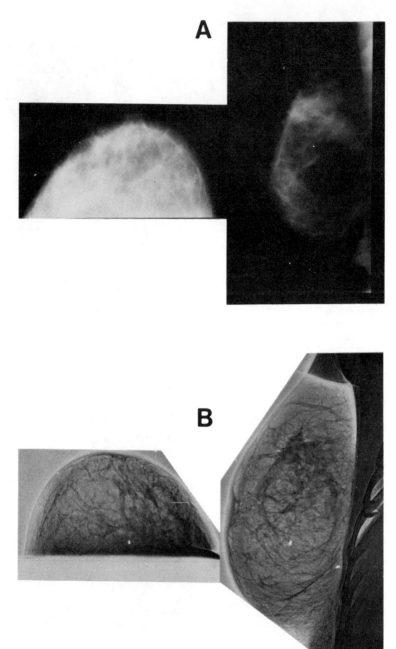

Fig. 7-3. A primary breast carcinoma is seen in the upper outer
quadrant of this 45 year old woman's left breast. It is
well-demarcated both mammographically (A) and xeroradiographically
(B). (Note: Craniocaudad view in 7-3B is mirror image; lesion
therefore appears medial instead of lateral).

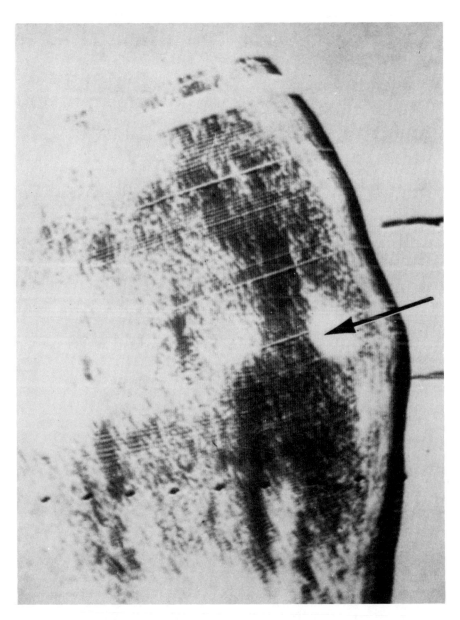

Fig. 7-4. Ultrasound image of right breast: Longitudinal sonogram
1cm. lateral to the nipple demonstrates cystic disease (arrow).

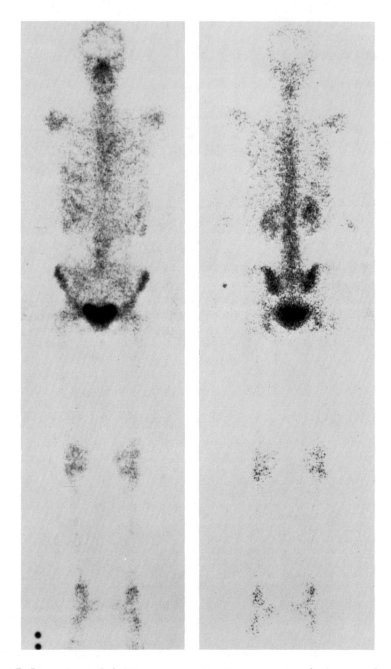

Fig. 7-5A. Serial bone scans over a seven month interval were similar to this, and failed to reveal any definite bony pelvic asymmetries.

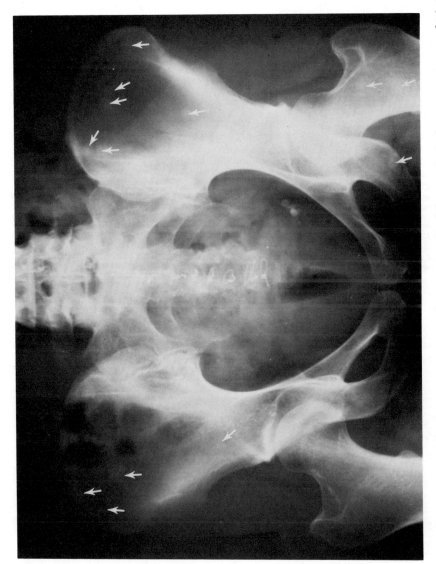

Fig. 7-5B. Pelvic roentgenogram at the onset of this period demonstrates multiple osteoblastic metastases involving the pelvis and proximal femur.

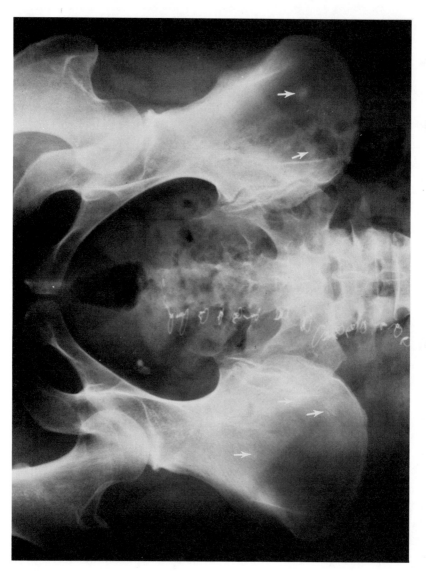

Fig. 7-5C. Despite the persistent absence of pelvic bone scan findings, obvious radiographic improvement is noted. Osteoblastic metastases, particularly in this location using the whole-body 5:1 reduction images, may cause false negative interpretations. Roentgenographic follow-up was clearly superior in this situation.

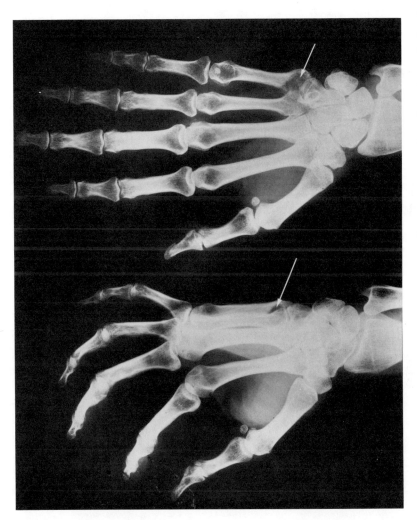

Fig. 7-6. Lytic metastasis to proximal right 5th metacarpal. Routine whole-body rectilinear scanning for bony metastases distal to the humerus has been unrewarding. Radiographic techniques may be more sensitive in detecting these uncommon sites. In the presence of localized bone pain, special camera views are advisable.

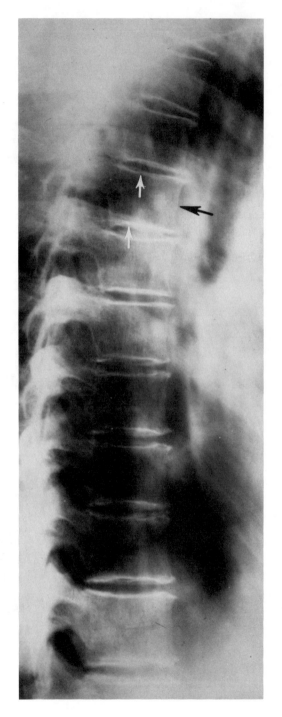

Fig. 7-7A. Metastatic bone disease can be more accurately assessed roentgenographically, following its initial detection by bone scan. Radiograph cf the dorsal spine reveals only minimal degenerative changes.

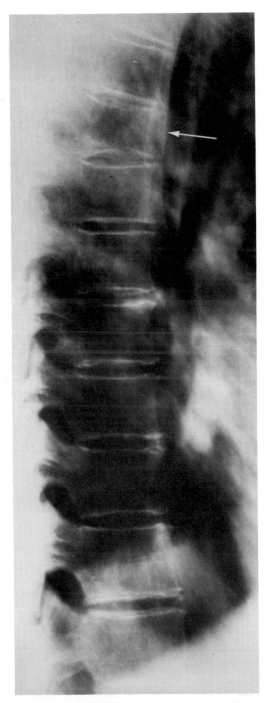

Fig. 7-7B. Three months following the first radiograph infraction
of the superior and inferior end plates of T-5 is noted.

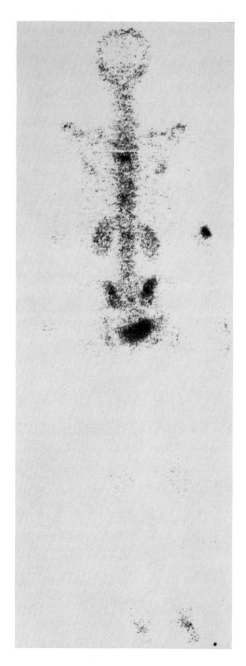

Fig. 7-7C. Posterior bone scan at the time of the Fig. 7-7B radiograph confirms this lesion and reveals additional suspicious tracer increases at T10-11, L-2 and the right sacroiliac joint.

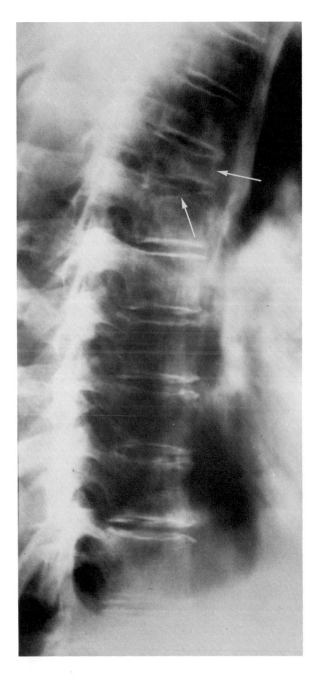

Fig. 7-7D. Follow-up radiograph five months later demonstrates disease progression with compression fracture of T-5 and depression of the T-6 superior end-plate.

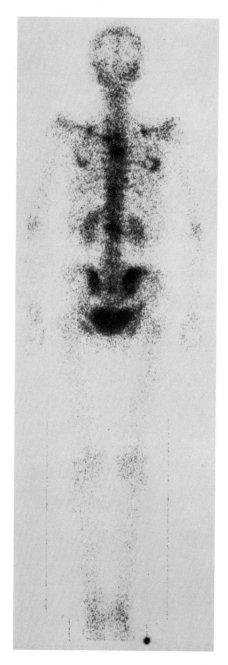

Fig. 7-7E. The bone scan, while more sensitive for detecting new metastatic disease, provides no further definition of disease progression at T5-6.

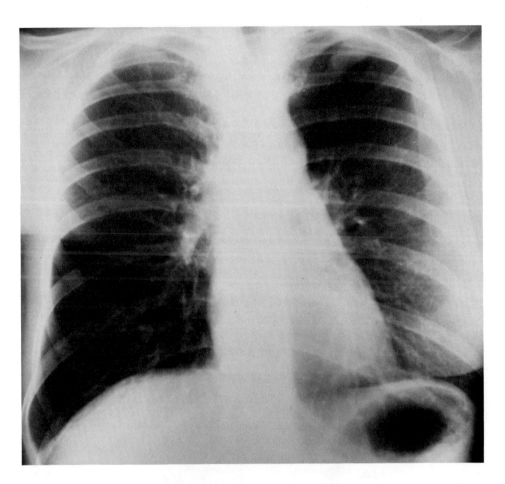

Fig. 7-8A. Chest radiograph in this post-right mastectomy patient demonstrated minimal fullness in the right hilum.

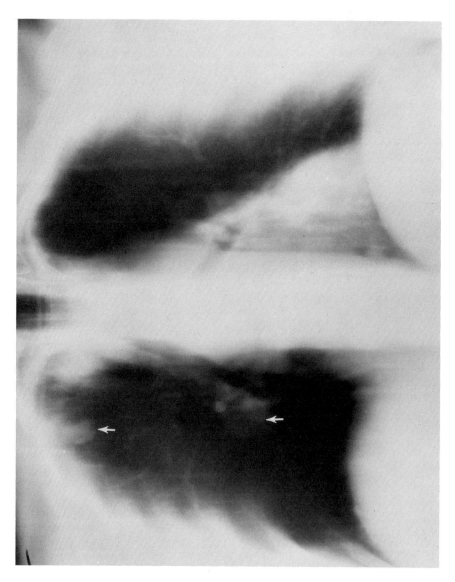

Fig. 7-8B. Full-lung tomography revealed a definite right hilar mass, in addition to an unsuspected right apical pulmonary metastasis. The value of tomography in the detection of secondary pulmonary involvement is apparent.

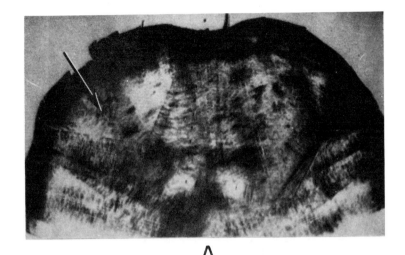

A

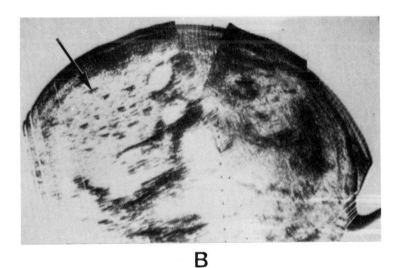

B

Fig. 7-9. Ultrasound images of the liver: Transverse sections 2 cms. beneath the xyphoid demonstrate the difficulty in hepatic evaluation with this technique. Note the similarity of the echo pattern in (A) hepatic metastases and (B) areas of post-inflammatory focal fibrosis. Arrow in right lobe identifies one of many abnormal areas.

References Chapter 7

1. Gershon-Cohen, J. Imperative changes in detection method
    for breast cancer. So Med J 64: 387, 1971.

2. Leger, J-L., Naimark, A.P., Beique, R.A., McFarlane, D.V.,
    Miller, S., Miller, A.B. Report of the "Ad Hoc" committee
    on mammography. J Canad Assn Radiol 25: 3, 1974.

3. Egan, R.L. Mammography and breast disease. Baltimore, Md.
    Williams and Wilkins, 1970.

4. Egan, R.L. Mammography. 2nd Ed. Springfield, Ill.,
    Charles C. Thomas, 1972

5. Wolfe, J.N. Xeroradiography of the breast. Springfield, Ill.,
    Charles C. Thomas, 1972.

6. Palmer, R.C., Egan, R.L., Tanner, B.K., Barnette, P.A.
    Absorbed dose in mammography using tungsten and moly-
    bdenum target tubes. Radiology 101: 697, 1971.

7. Dodd., G.D., Wallace, J.D., Freundlich, I.M., Marsh, L.,
    Zermino, A. Thermography and carcinoma of the breast.
    Cancer 23: 797, 1969.

8. Haberman, J.D. The role of thermography in breast cancer
    detection. Proc Natl Cancer Conf 6: 157, 1970.

9. Isard, H.J. Breast thermography after 4 years and 10,000
    studies. Amer J Roentgenol Radium Ther Nucl Med 115: 811, 1972.

10. Lilienfeld, A.M., Barnes, J.M., Barnes, R.B., Brasfield, R.,
    Connell, J.F., Diamond, E., Gershon-Cohen, J., Haberman, J.,
    Isard, H.J., Lane, W.Z., Lattes, R., Miller, J., Seaman, W.,
    Sherman, R. An evaluation of thermography in the detection
    of breast cancer: A cooperative pilot study. Cancer 24:
    1206, 1969.

11. Damascelli, B., Fossati, F., Livraghi, T., Severini, A.
    B-scan ultrasound exploration of neoplastic disease. Amer J
    Roentgenol Radium Ther Nucl Med, 105: 428, 1969.

12. DeLand, F. Modified technique of ultrasonography for detec-
    tion and differential diagnosis of breast lesions. Amer J
    Roentgenol Radium Ther Nucl Med 105: 446, 1969.

13.   Jellins, J., Kossoff, G., Buddee, F.W., Reeve, T.S. Ultra-
      sonic visualization of the breast. Med J Aust 1: 305, 1971.

14.   Wells, P.N.T., Evans, K.T. An immersion scanner for two-
      dimensional ultrasonic examination of the human breast.
      Ultrasonics 6: 220, 1968.

15.   Kossoff, G., Fry, E.K., Jellins, J. Average velocity of ultra-
      sound in the human female breast. J Acoust Soc Amer 53:
      1730, 1973.

16.   Abrams, H.L., Spiro, L.R., Goldstein, N. Metastasis in
      carcinoma. Analysis of 1,000 autopsied cases. Cancer
      3: 74, 1950.

17.   Carnett, J.B., Howell, J.C. Bone metastases in cancer
      of the breast. Ann Surg 91: 811, 1930.

18.   Freid, J.R., Goldberg, H. Frequency, clinical course and
      treatment of metastases from cancer of the breast. Amer J
      Roentgenol Radium Ther Nucl Med 50: 499, 1943.

19.   Lenz, M., Freid, J.R. Metastases to skeleton , brain and
      spinal cord from carcinoma of the breast and the effect of
      radiotherapy. Ann Surg 93: 278. 1931.

20.   Warren, S., Witham, E.M. Studies on tumor metastases: The
      distribution of metastases in cancer of the breast. Surg Gyn
      Obstet 57: 81, 1933.

21.   Turner, J.W., Jaffe, H.L. Metastatic neoplasms; A clinical and
      roentgenological study of involvement of skeleton and lungs.
      Amer J Roentgenol Radium Ther Nucl Med 43: 479, 1940.

22.   Rasmussen, S.N., Holm, H.H., Kristensen, J.K., Pedersen, J.F.,
      Hancke, S. Ultrasound in the diagnosis of liver disease.
      J Clin Ultrasound 1: 220, 1973.

23.   McCarthy, C.F., Davies, E., Wells, P.N., Ross, F.G.,
      Follett, D.H., Muir, K.M., Read, A.E. A comparison
      of ultrasonic and isotopic scanning in the diagnosis of
      liver disease. Brit J Rad 43: 100, 1970.

24.   McCarthy, C.F., Read, A.E., Ross, F.G.M., Wells, P.N.T.
      Ultrasonic scanning of the liver. Quart J Med 35: 517,
      1967.

25. Damascelli, B., Bonadonna, G., Roncoroni, L., Uslenghi, C.,
     Veronesi, V. Two-dimensional ultrasounds in liver diseases.
     JAMA 204: 963, 1968.

26. Leyton, B., Halpen, S., Leopold., G., Hagen, S. Correlation
     of ultrasound and colloid scintiscan studies of the normal
     and diseased liver. J Nucl Med 14: 27, 1973.

27. Taylor, K.J.W., Carpenter, D.A., McCready, V.R. Grey scale
     echography in the diagnosis of intrahepatic disease. J Clin
     Ultrasound 1: 284, 1973.

INDEX

THE L